The Clinical Smart Book

"The eyes can not see what the mind does not think."
- Phillip Zaret, M.D.

Raspberry Publishing Company

The Clinical Smart Book
A clinical guide to help transition from the basic sciences to clinical medicine
By Theodore T. Foley

Visit www.raspberrypublishing.com for order information.

Raspberry Publishing
Post Office Box 3822
York, PA 17042   U.S.A.
http://www.raspberrypublishing.com

Printed in the United States of America

Library of Congress Control Number: 2007929758

ISBN 978-0-9794071-0-9

Note: Much effort has been taken to assure that the information contained herein is correct. However, the author nor publisher guarantees the accuracy of the information in this publication. Furthermore, neither assumes any responsibility or liability for any consequences from application of the information in this book and makes no warranty, expressed or implied, with respect to the currency, completeness, or accuracy of the contents of this publication. This guide is not an authority on any of the subject matter presented herein. Most of this publication was written based upon my own personal experience, is intended to be educational and should not be assumed to be correct for direct patient care. Always seek patient management direction from a qualified physician such as your resident or attending. Multiple extensive, up-to-date, medical text books should be consulted before instituting any treatment for patient care.

Unless specifically noted otherwise, the information contained herein came from physicians and instructors of The Chicago Medical School as well as my own personal experience.

Preface

The transition from the basic sciences to clinical medicine can be overwhelming at first. The methods of learning are frankly, different. You must apply your knowledge, acquire and manage a large volume of new patient information, assimilate these and apply it to patient care. The experiences you have and the habits you form, during school will be the basis of your career, your foundation; don't squander your opportunity, you only go to school once.

The purpose of this guide is to help ease the transition from basic sciences to clinical medicine. The subject areas presented herein were all the things I wondered about when I was a student starting my clinical rotations. I often asked "What questions are relevant in the history when interviewing patients on this rotation? What parts of the physical exam should I focus on – given limited time?" Unfortunately I usually did not get a straight forward answer to these seemingly basic questions; all too often I received the "it depends" answer – which as a student gave me no place to start my foundation of learning. I have attempted to capture things that I learned on my rotations which seemed very relevant. Information which I wish I had acquired, before the rotation started. While the information in this book represents a small percent of the necessary information you will need to know, it is the *early necessary* information which will help you to quickly understand so you can get more out of your rotation.

This guide provides a starting point on areas to focus for the H&P while in each respective rotation. It provides tools/suggestions which help to organize patient data on a daily basis (you will be overwhelmed with patient data). The guide offers one method on how to approach common rudimentary skills which are the metal of all clinicians (e.g., Acid-base, EKGs, ABGs, etc.). There are always multiple approaches to clinical problems; I am giving you one method in this text. Eventually you will intuitively know what to do, what to ask, when to ask it, and how to mentally organize the pertinent information (by systems). Until that day comes, keep this guide in your coat pocket; pull it out as a memory jogger or as a brief orientation to the new rotation.

Keep in mind that this guide is not an authority on any of the subject matter presented herein. Most of this was gathered from my personal experiences with several references as well. Always seek patient management advice from an attending physician for patient care. It is very possible to get by without this guide, however as with any journey, having the right guide can make all the difference. I think reviewing the information presented herein, will significantly help in the transition from basic sciences to clinical medicine. Have fun and good luck!

Ted Foley, MD

iii

Table of Contents

Note: Patient Tracking Sheets for both Floor and ICU patients are available for free download and for modification, if so desired with Power Point, at www.raspberrypublishing.com.

General Advice

Recommended items to carry in your coat:
Maxwell's Quick Medical Reference, Tarascon pocket Pharmacopoeia, The Sanford Guide to Antimicrobial Therapy, Pen light, multiple black pens, Stethoscope, Reflex hammer, notepad or 5"x 8" note cards (scratch pad), many patient tracking sheets (see Medicine section) A pocket text like:

> *Pocket Medicine (Pocket Notebook)*, Marc S. Sabatine, M.D.
> *Clinician's Pocket Reference*, Leonard Gomella, Steven Haist
> *Medical Student's Pocket Reference*, Ken Bookstein, M.D.
> *Practical Guide to the Care of the Medical Patient*, Fred F. Ferri, M.D.
> *The Washington Manual of Medical Therapeutics*, Shubhada N. Ahya, et. al.
> *Tarascon Internal Medicine & Critical Care Pocketbook*, Robert J. Lederman, et.al
> Or similar text.

Note: Hospitals provide things like the otoscope, ophthalmoscope and sphygometers.

Sage Advice
1. The most important task during your M3 year should be to decide your profession. You have to apply somewhere the end of your third year. You should decide by the winter break, M3 year.

2. The sequence of M3 year is important for several reasons. Senior year, students often do an "audition rotation" at a residency where they would like to match. To do this usually requires having passed (verifiable through transcript, which could take ~10 weeks after the clerkship) the M3 clerkship in your field of interest, prior to application. Also, you might need a letter of recommendation (this is rare) just to apply to do that senior year rotation. However, if you have a choice, it is better to not elect to do your area of interest as your first rotation M3 year, but to hone your skills by taking other clerkships first. You'll feel like a fumbling buffoon early in M3 year, especially for your first rotation. You don't want to do poorly in the field you wish to pursue for residency.

3. M3/M4 year timeline...
February: start applying to do your "audition rotation" (only if you plan to...it's optional, but often recommended). At this point you should have somewhat of a list of residency programs you are interested in applying. (Consider fellowship possibilities, quality of program, cost of living & outside of work social activities).
March: start writing your personal statement (I revised my PS about 25 times before submitting it to ERAS-see note below. Some people will submit 2 or 3 personal statements to ERAS).
August: enter ERAS application into the internet.
October – January: Interviews. Some programs don't give you a choice and will invite you for a single day; most give you a choice of dates to select from. Think about this in planning M4 electives; some rotations will be more forgiving than others regarding allowing travel time for interviews.
February: Second or third week, submit your final 'rank list'.
March: Match day.

Note: ERAS is the internet residency application www.aamc.org. NRMP is the internet computer program/algorithm that matches all the medical students to residencies www.nrmp.org

1

4. Maximize your learning. You will spend 30-120 minutes per day M3/M4 year driving to your rotations. Listen to tapes/CDs of medical stuff (library) while sitting in traffic; you'd be surprised how much stuff sinks in while you're driving. Read something everyday.

5. M4 electives:
    a. Take an ICU rotation to learn ABGs, ventilators and gain confidence for internship. You will learn more during those four weeks than you will learn in four months of other rotations.
    b. Take a Cardiology rotation to gain EKG confidence.
    c. Take a Radiology rotation to learn how to read films.
    d. Learn ACLS; everyone will have to use it during residency.

Some remaining thoughts…

- Treat the patient, not the monitors/labs (this is a very profound statement; everyone makes this mistake, don't let it happen to you.)

- Vital signs are vital for a reason. Always personally make sure the vitals you are reporting are accurate. (90% of problems can be picked up from vitals, the CBC and BMP).

- One last thought: What will your contribution be?

Presentation: IS VIP DNR

Intro
Subj.
Vitals
I + O
PE (pertinent)
Drug list
New Study Results
Review of chart (nurse notes, etc)
* Assessment + Plan *

Medicine

History
Name
Date and Time
Demographic info.: age, gender, ethnic
Source of Hist./Referral: family, friend...
Chief Complaints (CC): Patient's why at the hospital
History of Present Illness: (OLD QIRE ASAP-F)
symptoms as: onset, location, duration, quality, intensity, radiation, exacerbation, alleviation, setting it occurs, assoc. manifestations, past history, freq
    Current Medications: dose, freq., duration, reason, compliance (any pill/herb)
    Allergies: w/specific rxn
Past Medical History:
    Child Illnesses: Viruses
    Adult Illnesses:
        Medical (diabetes, HTN, Asthma, HIV, HEP B, Hosp.)
        Surgical (date, indication, outcome)
        OB GYN (menstrual hist, birth control, # of partners)
        Psychiatric (dates, diag., treatments)
        Accidents, Injuries & Transfusions
Family History: age, health & Illnesses (DM, CVD, COPD, Kidney, Bleeding, CA)
Preventive Health History: Age related screening, immunizations, TB tests, pap smears, mammograms, colonoscopy, PSA levels, DM testing, last doctor's office visit
Social History: tobacco products, alcohol, drugs, marital stat, relationships, persons at home, occupation, hobbies, exercise, diet, caffeine beverages
Travel History:
Review of Systems (ROS):

General
state of health, fever, chills, usual weight, change of weight, weakness, fatigue, sweats, radiation exposure, headaches, pulse feeling from head

Head
dizziness, headaches, pain, fainting, history of head injury, stroke, visual disturbances, scalp changes, lumps, itching

Eyes
use of eyeglasses, current vision, change of vision, diplopia - double vision, excessive tearing, pain, recent eye examinations, photophobia-pain when looking at light, unusual sensations like [floaters, scintillations-luminous wavy patch in visual field, scotmas-island like blind spot in visual field, teichopsia- scintillating scotoma in eyes usu assoc with migraines], discharge, redness, infections, injuries, sudden blindness, glaucoma - inc intraocular press, cataracts - Opacity of the lens

Ears
hearing impairment, use of hearing aid, discharge, dizziness, pain, tinnitus - ringing in ears, infections, vertigo, earache

Nose
epistaxis - nosebleeds, infections, stuffiness, itching, allergy, rhinorrhea – watery discharge, freq of colds, nasal obstruction, sinus area pain

Mouth & Throat
condition of teeth, last dental appointment, condition of gums, bleeding gums, burning tongue, nasal tone, hoarseness, voice changes, postnasal drip, taste disturbance, swallowing difficulties, tooth pain, dentures fit well?

Neck
lumps, goiter, dysphagia – difficulty swallowing, pain on movement, dizziness on turning neck, tenderness of glands, history of swollen glands, thyroid trouble, stiffness

Chest
cough, sputum, hemoptysis - coughing blood, pain, SOB, wheezing, sputum prod (quality & appearance), pleurisy - inflammation of the pleura, bronchitis, wheezing, last x-ray

Breasts
lumps, discharge, pain, tenderness, discharge, self-examinations? last mammogram?

Skin
rashes [bleeding from lesions, scaly lesions, ulcerations, skin breaks], pruritis – sever itching, dryness, changes in: [skin color (jaundice, pallor), texture, nail texture], lumps, moles, use of hair dyes, flakiness/redness around [nose, forehead, patches of elbows, knees], changes in current skin markings, dermatographism – raised wheal produced by gentle scratching, nail changes

Cardiac
chest pain radiation, chest tightness, heaviness, angina, high blood pressure, edema, murmurs, hx of rheumatic fever, palpitations - rapid, throbbing pulsation; fluttering of the heart, dyspnea on exertion (DOE) - SOB with activity, paradoxical nocturnal dyspnea (PND) - sudden SOB while sleeping, orthopnea – SOB in any psn except erect psn, orthodeoxia – decreased oxygen concentration while upright (assoc. w/ infection of PCP or hepatopulmonary syn), last ECG (or other heart tests such as stress test or ECHO)

Gastrointestinal
appetite (excessive hunger/thirst), nausea, vomiting, constipation, diarrhea, heartburn, indigestion, dysphagia – difficulty swallowing [liquids, solids], odynophagia - pain upon swallowing, abdominal pain, stool change? [color, caliber/size, consistency], melenia - black tarry stool, hematochezia - stool with purple/red color, mucus in stool, bowel movements[last one?, frequency], hematemesis - vomiting of blood, rectal[bleeding, pain], laxative or antacid use, excessive belching, food intolerance, change in abdominal size, hemorrhoids, infections, jaundice, urine change in color, abdomen tenderness, what happens when you eat fatty foods?

Urinary
Frequency, urgency, incontinence – leaking, hesitancy – involuntary delay in starting, polyuria, dysuria – pain while urinating, nocturia - awaking to night urinate, hematuria - blood in urine, urination[color, odor, frequency, excessive, burning], infections, stones, enuresis – involuntary discharge of urine, nocturnal enuresis - bed wetting, flank pain

Male Genitalia

lesions, pain, discharge, impotence - weakness in maintaining erection, sores, scrotal masses, testicular pain, lumps in groin that stick out, freq of intercourse, ability to enjoy sexual relations, contraception?, hx of sex transmitted diseases, priapism – abnormal, painful and continued erection

Female Genitalia

lesions, itching, discharge, STDs/treatment, intercourse[dyspareunia – pain during intercourse, freq., ability to enjoy], fertility problems, bulges in groin, menarche – initial age of first menstrual period [age @, interval, duration of, amount of flow, date of last, bleeding between], dysmenorrhea - pain upon, menorrhagia – excessive but regular menstrual bleeding, metrorrhagia – irregular vaginal bleeding, menometrorrhagia – irregular or excessive menstrual bleeding], menopause - age of, pregnancies and complications, miscarriages/abortions, birth control, post menopause bleeding, DES - diethylstilbestrol exposure(daughters will have reproductive track problems when their moms' took it to prevent abortions during pregnancy)

Musculoskeletal

weakness, paralysis, stiffness, limited movement, joint pain/stiffness, back pain, radiating, only in the morning, muscle cramps, deformities, tenderness, swelling of joint as a child

Neurologic

fainting, dizziness, blackouts, syncope - to pass out, numbness, tingling, burning, tremors, loss of memory, mood changes[depressed, anxious, rage, too happy, nervousness], speech disorders, gait unsteady, general behavioral change, loss of consciousness, hallucinations [visual, auditory, olfactory], disorientation, weakness, suicidal ideation

Psychiatric

mood, anxiety, depression, tension, memory (see Psychiatric section of this book)

Endocrine

heat or cold intolerance, polyuria - excessive urine, polydipsia - excessive thirst, polyphagia – gluttony (eating abnormally large amounts), change in libido, weight loss/gain, excessive sweating, salt craving

Hematologic

Bleeding, easy bruising, weakness, pallor, fatigue, swollen glands, blood spots on skin, how long to stop bleeding, gums bleeding, anemia hx, sneezing, burning or watery eyes, HIV

Vascular

Pain in [legs, calves, thighs, hips while walking or gluteal pain], swelling of legs, varicose veins, thrombophlebitis- thrombus causes inflammation of a vein, coolness of extremity, loss of hair on legs, discoloration of extremity, ulcers, claudication - calf pain only when walking, clots

Obstetrical History   GxPxxxx (Gravida/Para)

-Gravida - # times preg with child
-Para – 1. term live births (a viable infant [>500g or >20 weeks] regardless of whether the infant is alive at birth 2. spontaneous abortion 3. induced termination 4. # living children
-delivery problems?

Physical Examination Checklist

Key: [optional] *Ask the patient these questions*
Supplies: a cup of water, BP cuff, watch, card to cover eyes, eye chart, Ophthalmoscope, Otoscope, Tuning forks (512 Hz & 128 Hz), stethoscope, tongue depressor, cotton ball, Q-tip

Introduction: **Wash hands**

<u>Vital Signs</u> (most important part of the exam)
Blood pressure (L & R) Sitting (heart level) [Supine, Standing]
Radial Pulse (>15 sec) Sitting [(L & R) Supine, Standing]
Respiratory rate (>15 sec)

<u>Head & Sinuses</u>
Observe Scalp (size, shape, contours)
Palpate Scalp (a. hair texture/quantity
 b. scaliness, lesions, lumps
 c. sweep for lumps, tender areas)
Fontal Sinus **Palpate (L & R)** [tenderness?]
Maxillary Sinus **Palpate (L & R)** [tenderness?]
[Transillumination] [Inspect face for symmetry, masses, and expressions]

<u>Nodes & Thyroid</u>
Palpate lymph nodes:
Preauricular (front of ear)
Post auricular (behind ear)
Occipital (base of skull)
Anterior cervical (in front of SCM)
Post cervical (behind SCM)
Supra clavicular (above collarbone)
Tonsillary (angle of jaw)
Submandibular (between tonsillar & submental)
Submental (under chin)

Thyroid; Observe swallowing (offer water)
Thyroid; Palpate (from behind)
Thyroid; Palpate w/ swallowing (offer water)

<u>Eyes</u>
CN 2
Visual acuity (only L & only R) (14" away; note glasses/contacts)
Visual fields (only L & only R) (test each eye, of quadrant separately)
 Can you see my fingers? **(stand 12" away)**
 patient close R/student L
 finger wiggle test 45°, -45°, 135°, -135°
 switch closed eyes; repeat finger wiggle test
Check for convergence (arm's length to 6")

CN 3, 4, 6
head still; follow finger: 'H' - Right, up, down - Left, up, down
(must test all 6 cardinal positions)

6

CN 7 (upper div)
Close eyes very tight - against resistance
Inspect each eye: lid, cornea, conjunctiva [eyebrows, lacrimal apparatus]

CN 2, 3
pupillary responses: direct response & consensual (L & R)
[check for corneal reflections; alignment & symmetry]

Psn patient at a *comfortable height* for examiner
Ophthalmoscope
        (R eye, R hand, patient's R eye)
        (L eye, L hand, patient's L eye)
[arteries/veins; optic disc/cup]
[findings: hemorrhages, scars, exudates]

Ear
Whisper test (2ft) or finger rub (10cm)
Inspect the external ear (front, pull to look behind)
Otoscope exam (pull the ear back)
[Tympanic membrane (perforation, inflammation, mobility, ossicles)]
[external auditory meatus]

Rinne test (512 Hz) (L & R)
    place on mastoid process; ask the patient 'tell me when you don't hear sound.'
    At that point, move the fork in front of ear canal; 'tell me when you don't hear sound.'
    (Then, listen to see if you can hear the sound)
[Conductive loss: BC>AC or BC=AC] [Sensorineural loss: AC>BC (which is normal)]

Weber test (512 Hz) (on skin, center of top of head)
    Ask the patient **'where do you hear the sound?'**
[hear on side of air conductive loss or opposite the side of sensorineural loss (bone conduction)]

Nose
Patient: close one passage; sniff (L & R) (testing patency of each passage)

Mouth and Throat
Inspect: lips, gums, teeth, tongue, and oral mucosa
Inspect: posterior pharynx (use tongue blade & light)
    (Ask patient to *breath only through your mouth*)
[soft palate, pillars, tonsils] [*Observe elevation of palate "ah" (CN 10)*]

CN 12   **protrude tongue directly out & move side to side**
CN 5   **bite down: feel masseter muscles**
CN 7   **show teeth (CN 7 lower division)**
CN 11   **rotate head against resistance (L & R)**
            shrug shoulders against resistance (L & R)

Lungs & Thorax
Percussion: (compare L then R) posterior   3, 6, 9 (intercostals spaces)
Auscultate: the same (*'breath through an open mouth'*)
[Auscultate: 1. vesicular - insp 100%/exp 33% [soft & low pitch]
                2. bronchial - insp 100%/exp 120% [louder & higher pitch]
                3. crackles (sounds like 'popping')
If abnormal,
Bronchophony (say "99"; normal: muffled & indistinct; abnormal: louder clearer)
Egophony (say "ee"; normal: "E"; abnormal: "ay")
Whispered pectoriloqy (whisper "1-2-3"; normal: faint; abnormal: louder, clearer)]

Percussion: (compare L then R) anterior   3 [5, 7]
Auscultate: the same (*'breath through an open mouth'*)
[Inspect chest: audible breathing, deformities (excavatum, carinaturn), dyspnea respiratory
excursion, asymmetry, intercostals retraction, accessory muscle use]

[Palpate: 1. Chest wall & sternum: tenderness
                2. Tactile fremitus (normal: feel voice sounds)
                (front & back (L & R; around the scapula))
                3. Expansion (breaths in: feel for unilateral expansion)
                4. Axillae for adenopathy (tenderness)]

[Diaphragmatic excursion (diff. between resonant vs. dull line; on back; normal 5-6 cm)]
[full inspiration] [full expiration]

Breast Exam part I
Ask patient to: *lower gown* so that both breasts are visible & arms *above head*
Inspect: for dimpling, contour changes & skin discolor
Ask patient to: *Place hands on hips and press inward*
Inspect: for dimpling
Ask patient to: *Put gown back on*
Palpate the axillary nodes:
        anterior axillary fold
        posterior axillary fold
        proximal humerus
        deep axillary vault
Ask the patient to *lie down* on the table

Breast Exam Part II
Degown one side at a time; Ask patient to *raise arm* above the head
(use your middle 3 fingers, R hand)
Start at the top sternal side of breast, palpate each spot in light, medium & firm
pressure (fingers must not lose contact with skin) use 'strip' technique down, up, down,
up, etc. (repeat for other breast)

Heart
Still supine
Raise trunk/head/neck to: Measure jugular venous pressure
(straight edge & ruler)
(Or if not present, view the jugular vein pulsation)

patient *upright or supine*
[Inspect (point of max impulse)]
Palpate (for: tenderness, crepitation, heave, apical pulse, and thrill)
      R2 aortic   (near center)
      L2/3 pulmonic   (near center)
      L4/5 tricuspid   (near the sternal edge)
      L5 mitral/apical (midclavicular line)
[Percuss (for: dullness to assess size)]

Auscultate (for: rhythm, S1, S2, Murmurs, clicks, friction rubs)
      Diaphragm (all 4 areas)
      Bell (all 4 areas)
          R2 aortic
          L2/3 pulmonic
          L4/5 tricuspid
          5 mitral/apical
[valsalva, squatting (helps to ID sys murmurs; splitting of S1/S2)]

Pulses
Ask patient to hold breath
Auscultate carotid artery (bruits)
Palpate: (note quality 'full, bounding, weak', regularity)
  (L & R) carotid (medial and below jaw)
  (L & R) femoral
  (L & R) political
  (L & R) post tibial (posterior to the medial malleolus)
  (L & R) dorsal pedis

Abdomen
Ask the patient to *lie down*
[Inspect   (color, contour, venous patterns, pulsations)]
Auscultate each quadrant (listen for bowel sounds)
        [Renal arteries (bruits)] [Aorta (bruits)]

Palpate   (for: masses, tenderness)
        each quadrant (gently then firm)
        Spleen (inhale/push up & in/exhale)

Percuss liver   (R of midline & midclavicular)
Palpate liver edge (inhale/exhale)
[Special maneuvers:
Liver size   (Auscultate over liver and scratch lightly abdomen moving toward liver)
Ascites   (lye on back: dull around a central tympanic area)
Shifting dullness (lye on side: dull on bottom, tympanic on top)
Fluid wave   (lye on back: press on midline, tap one side and feel other side)
Murphy's sign: gallbladder
Appendicitis:
  McBurney's point: (33% from sup ant iliac spine)
  Rousing's sign: (push on L, feel pain on R)
  Obturator: (rotate foot out, or bend knee and rotate foot medial)
  Psoas, Rectal, Pelvic]

Musculoskeletal Examination
Ask the patient to *sit up*
Inspect, ask the patient to:

Fingers
(spread fingers)   **Extension of fingers (inspect palmar & dorsal side)** [feel for nodules]
(make fists)   **Flexion (inspect)** (redness & swelling)
                        Watch finger flexion & extension
Wrist
  Extend
  Flex

Elbow
  Inspect elbows (bursa swelling)
  Supinate (Flex & Extend)
  Pronate (Flex & Extend)
Stand *behind* the patient (*gown untied & open in back*)

10

<u>Shoulder</u>
 flexion (<u>arms forward</u>, then over head)
 external rotation (hands on neck, elbows back)
 internal rotation(arms in back, high up)
[with hand on the shoulder - feeling for crepitus]
Ask patient to *lie down*

Inspect the quadriceps muscle

<u>Hip</u>
Range of Motion
 flexion (I move foot towards thorax)
 external/internal rotation
 (thigh is ⊥; shin is parallel; rotate med/lat)

<u>Knee</u>
Inspection (atrophy of quad, fossae (medial & lateral), shape & size of patella, skin lesions?)
Range of Motion
 Flexion (swelling?)
 Extension
[Abduction stress test, Adduction stress test, Anterior Drawer Sign, Posterior Drawer Sign]

<u>Ankle & Foot</u>
Inspect (swelling or redness)
Range of motions
 dorsiflexion
 plantarflexion

[inversion of heel (subtalar), eversion of heel (subtalar), inversion of transverse tarsal joint, eversion of transverse tarsal joint]

Inspect: plantar surface, midfoot, toes
[Assess straight leg raising]

<u>Neck</u>
 flexion (chin to chest)
 extension (look to ceiling)
 rotation (chin on shoulder, both)
 lateral bending (ear to shoulder, both)

Ask the patient to *stand* (stand *behind* the patient, *gown untied*)
Observe the alignment of the knees, heels, and feet

I will place me hands on your hips to hold your gown on and to prevent you from falling in the following tasks.

The Spine
Range of Motion
>**Thoracolumbar (bend to the L & R)**
>**Lumbar (bend to touch toes)**
>[Schober test - standing measure 10 cm; flexion 14 cm is normally seen]
>**Lumbar extension (bend backwards)**
>**kidney tap test; costovertebral angles; any pain?**

Neurologic Evaluation
Romberg Test
>(stand, eyes <u>open</u> for **15 sec**) (look for sway) *I won't let you fall*
>(stand, eyes <u>closed</u> for **15 sec**) (look for sway)

walk away (observe gait & sensorium)
walk back on tip toes
walk away, on heels
walk back, heel-to-toe (tandem gait; like walking a line)
Ask patient to *have a seat*

Drift test (arms in front, eyes closed, palms up, 15 sec)
Muscle strength testing (I'm pushing/pulling)
Ask patient to resist my push/pull
>**Grip**   (C7, 8, T1)
>**Deltoid**   **(I push on abducted arms)**
>**Biceps**   (C5, 6)
>**Triceps**   (C6, 7, 8)
>**Hip flexor**   (L2, 3, 4) **(raise knee)**
>**Plantar flex foot**   (S1) **('push')**
>**Dorsiflex foot**   (L4, 5) **('pull')**

DTRs
position *arm in patient's lap*
>**Biceps (palpate w/finger, strike)**
>**Brachioradialis (radius, 2" above wrist)**
>**Triceps (posterior)**
>**Patellar**
>**Achilles (slightly dorsiflex the foot)**
>**Babinski (heel/lateral/at ball turn medially)**

(Positive sign: dorsiflex big toe & fanning of the other toes; Normal: toes plantar flex)
[Pathological Reflexes: (lesion in the corticospinal tract)
Chaddock: Scratch the lateral malleolus, then along the dorsum of the foot
Openheimer: knuckles to the skin of the tibia and slide them down toward the ankle]

Cerebellar function test:
finger-to nose coord. (nose to my finger to nose (move my finger))
[Heel to skin (heel on contralateral knee, move down shin to big toe)]
[Dysdiadochokinesis: (inability to: tap foot, alt, against my hand as fast as possible)]

Sensation
Demonstrate sharp vs. dull (light touch - cotton ball; sharp - broken end of Q-tip (wooden))
Ask patient to *close their eyes*
upper extremities, lower extremities, trunk

Position Sense
Big toe: **show up/down**, then *close eyes*
test up vs. down - patient states 'up' or 'down'

Vibration [128 HZ]
demo - while patient watches on a bony prominence
test (close eyes, each big toe or each ankle, patient states when vibration stops)

Test each tibia, medial malleolus, or dorsum for edema (3-5 sec press)

SCALES
Pulse: scale of 0-4
    4=bounding
    3=full, increased
    2=expected
    1=diminished, barely palpable
    0=absent

Edema: Scale of 1+ to 4+
    1+ = 2mm depression left in skin
    2+ = 4mm depression
    3+ = 6mm depression
    4+ = 8mm depression

Muscle Strength: Scale 0-5+
    5+ = Full strength against resistance
    4+ = Good strength, examiner can "overcome" the patient's strength
    3+ = Able to lift limb against gravity but not against any resistance
    2+ = Able to move limb in a plane but not against gravity
    1+ = spontaneous fasciculations
    0= no movement

Deep tendon reflexes: Scale 0-4+
    0 = No response
    1+= Sluggish, diminished
    2+= Active and/or expected response
    3+= More brisk than expected, slightly hyperactive
    4+= Brisk, hyperactive with intermittent clonus

Note: the patient tracking sheets are very valuable for the Medicine rotation, available for free download at www.raspberrypublishing.com

References: Bickley, LS. Bates' Guide to Physical Examination and History Taking, 7th edition, Lippincott Williams & Wilkins, Philadelphia, 1999.

Notes

Surgery

(Acute Abdomen H&P)

History

CC:

HPI: (OLD QIRE ASAP-F)
onset, location, duration, quality(1-10), intensity, radiation, exacerbation, alleviation, setting it occurs, assoc. manifestations, past history, freq
   Meds: (steroids?)
   Allergies: w/specific rxn
PMH:(?DM, CVD, HTN, Asthma, HIV, HEP B, thyroid, Hospitalizations.)
PSH: (date, indication, outcome)
FH: mom, dad, siblings(? DM, CVD, COPD, Kidney, Bleeding, CA)
SH: tobacco products, alcohol, drugs
ROS: (Abdominal pain - high yield)
F/Chills/N/V/D/constipation?
Dysuria/Frequency/Urgency/flank pain?
Anorexia?
Last: BM?, meal?, pain in relation to meals?
Change in bowel habits?
LMP?, vaginal discharge?
Melena?, hematochezia?, hematemesis?

PE
Vitals: Tmax, Tnow, P , BP, RR, O_2sat (vitals are the most important – ensure accuracy)
General: how is the patient in bed? (motionless=peritonitis, restless=nephrolithiasis)
HEENT: JVD, Bruits, thryromegaly
CV: S1S2, RRR, murmur
Chest: crackles, rhonchi, wheezing
Abdomen: (psn the pt flat with abdominal muscles relaxed, proper draping)
   Inspection: scars, distention
   Auscultation: bowel sounds, bruits, size of liver
   Palpation: soft/rigid, tender, rebound, guarding, CVA tenderness, size of liver
   Percussion: liver, spleen size
Pelvic: motion tenderness
Rectal: motion tenderness, occult stool blood
Ext: edema, pulses, bruits

Labs: CBC w/diff, CHEM10, amylase, lipase, type & screen, UA, LFTs, Beta-hcg
Tests: CXR, AXR/KUB, CT

Ddx:
RUQ: cholecystitis, choledocholithiasis, cholangitis, pyelonephritis, nephrolithiasis, hepatitis, hepatic abscess, liver tumor, PUD, perforated ulcer, pancreatitis, gastritis, appendicitis, pneumonia, PE, MI, pericarditis, PTX

LUQ: pancreatitis, GERD, PUD, perforated ulcer, gastritis, splenic rupture/dz, abscess, hepatitis, hepatic abscess, liver tumor, pneumonia, PE, MI, PTX, pericarditis, pyelonephritis, nephrolithiasis, Boerhaave's syn, Mallory-Weiss tear, splenic artery aneurysm

LLQ: diverticulitis, SBO, sigmoid volvulus, perforated colon, colon CA, IBD (crohn's dz/ ulcerative colitis), ectopic pregnancy, ovarian torsion, testicular torsion, tubo-ovarian abscess, cancer of cervix/uterus/ovary

RLQ: appendicitis, diverticulitis, Meckel's diverticulum, intussusception, and all LLQ possibilities

Non-surgical causes of abdominal pain
UTI, Gastroenteritis (pain after vomiting), pregnancy, DKA, sickle cell, mesenteric lymphadenitis, porphyria, PID, mittelschmerz, endometriosis, fibroids, kidney stone, pyelonephritis, hepatitis, pancreatitis, pneumonia, MI, C. difficile, ovarian cyst

HIV: CMV, TB, Kaposi's, lymphoma, mycobacterium avium

(ROS: lower yield – Surgery in general)
HEENT: Recent upper respiratory tract infection? Sore throat? Cough?
GI: antacid use/NSAID use, rectal bleeding?
Cardiac: angina, palpitations, dyspnea on exertion (DOE), paradoxical nocturnal dyspnea (PND) - sudden SOB while sleeping, orthopnea – SOB in any psn except erect psn, last ECG (or other heart tests)
Male Genitalia: testicular pain, lumps in groin that stick out
Female Genitalia: discharge, STDs/treatment, intercourse [dyspareunia – pain during intercourse, frequency, bulges in groin, menstrual period [interval, duration of, amount of flow, date of last, bleeding between], dysmenorrhea - pain upon, menorrhagia – excessive but regular menstrual bleeding, metrorrhagia – irregular vaginal bleeding, menometrorrhagia – irregular or excessive menstrual bleeding], birth control
Hematologic: bleeding, easy bruising, weakness, pallor, fatigue
Vascular: Pain in [legs, calves, thighs or hips while walking], swelling of legs, varicose veins, thrombophlebitis - thrombus causes inflammation of a vein, coolness of extremity, loss of hair on legs, discoloration of extremity, ulcers, claudication - calf pain only when walking, clots

Surgery pre-Rounds
(always present vitals first)

SOAP Note: (floor patients; for ICU pts see ICU section)
S: how does the pt feel? N/V/F/C? passed any gas? BM's? pain? chest pain? SOB? pain medicine helping? appetite? sleep last night? bleeding?

O: Tmax, Tnow, Pulse, BP, RR, O_2%, I/O, Fingerstick blood glucose
I/O: urine output last 24 or 8hrs, IVFs, oral intake, stool, tube outputs
MS: A&Ox3, distress
CV:
Resp:
Abd: BS? (be gentle), NT? distended? incision: erythema? bleeding? (look under dressing after 48 hrs) dehiscence?
Ext: edema? Homan's sign (dorsiflex foot & squeeze calf gently, if pain= +)? Were SCDs on when you can in the room? Or TEDs?
Note: Incisions, drains, lines, ostomy sites (red? swollen? discharge?) Do not look at wound until 48 hours after surgery.

Labs: current labs. (know trends)
X-ray: Results of any imaging studies
Meds: Know current meds. (esp. antibiotics and day# of that abx).

A/P: # yo POD #1 s/p procedure…

Pre-Op Note
1) Pre-op diagnosis
2) Procedure planned
3) Indications for procedure
4) Lab results
5) CXR
6) EKG
7) Blood - type and crossed for 2 U PRBC
8) Orders – NPO, abx, skin/colon prep
9) Permit - Procedure described to patient, along with risks and benefits explained, consent signed, witnessed, and in chart.

Operative Note (PPP SAFE DCCS)
1) Pre-op Dx
2) Post-op Dx
3) Procedure
4) Surgeons
5) Anesthesia
6) Findings
7) EBL (estimated blood loss) - type and location, also: Fluids-IV and urine output
8) Drains
9) Complications
10) Condition - Pt tolerated procedure well, sent to recovery room in stable condition.
11) Specimens
Reference:
   Blackbourne, LH. Surgical Recall. Lippincott Williams & Wilkins, Baltimore, 2002.

Notes

Emergency Medicine

Emergency Medicine is exactly that, emergent. You have to think about the acute problems that will hurt the patient in the **short term**. You're trying to triage the patient. You want to gather enough information to get the patient in front of the physician who can most help that patient the fastest. *You're not there to solve all the patient's problems.* Dr. Phillip Zaret, an amazing surgeon at Mt. Sinai Chicago, says "The eyes can not see what the mind does not think." Meaning, you have to think about what to look for, or you might note find what is there. You have to know what medical conditions the patient has in order to correctly conduct the history, physical exam, ordering of tests, and to know who to consult. Emergency medicine is difficult. Often many physicians are retrospectively very critical of seemingly strange things that took place in the ER regarding a particular patient. Think about the ER physician's perspective. Many concurrent things are going on in the ER. ER physicians have to be very insightful, quick, and able to multitask very serious patient situations. They are forced to make decisions with very limited information, often when daytime resources (such as family) are not available to help with these decisions.

The history and physical should be focused around the above thoughts. Your presentation to the attending should be succinct. Try to present the entire patient in less than 1-2 minutes (including what you would like to do). Relevant positive and negative, don't mention anything superfluous. Occasionally more time presenting is warranted, occasionally. The H&P is the same as for Internal Medicine (see that section), just keep it short and focused on the acute problem. The acute problem. The acute problem. (reiterated for clarity & emphasis).

You can make a difference in patient care and learn a lot by doing several things. You should try to do as many procedures as possible such as placing IV lines, draw blood, suture wounds, placing Foley catheters, arterial blood gases, splinting fractures, lumbar spinal taps, rectal exams, and pelvic exams. Of course always write procedure notes when you've completed a procedure. Know where equipment is located; look around the ER during breaks. When that trauma comes in and they send you to get a Foley Catheter kit (or anything else), do you know where the kits are kept? Look at the packages, noting sizes and what is in each kit. Continually check in on your patient and notify the resident if anything has changed (is your asthma patient, who was really having a hard time breathing 30 min ago, now 'sleepy' and not having difficulty breathing anymore? Or is that asthma patient crashing?) Get involved in the traumas, if possible. Help the staff in any way possible, no matter how trivial it may seem. For example, putting pressure on a patient's cricoid cartilage during intubation (the Sellick maneuver), may allow that resident to intubate the patient and prevent aspiration, otherwise the patient might get a really bad aspiration pneumonia or possibly die!

The small pocket-sized NMS book *Emergency Medicine* by Biddinger, Adler, Plantz, Sterns, and Gossman is a nice practical supplement to use while seeing patients during the rotation.

Below are suture guidelines which should help with you to determine suture type, size, and removal times.

Location	Suture Size	Days until Removal
Scalp	3-O or 4-O (or staple)	7-10
Face	6-O	3-5
Trunk	4-O or 5-O	7-10
Arm	4-O or 5-O	10-12
Leg	3-O or 4-O	12-14
Joints	4-O or 5-O	14
Sub-Q or fascia	3-O or 4-O	

Nonabsorbable Sutures : Silk, Nylon, Prolene
Absorbable Sutures: Chromic Gut, Vicryl, PDS

Note: see *Template* section for Procedure note format.

Reference: The NMS book *Emergency Medicine* by Biddinger, Adler, Plantz, Sterns, and Gossman
Special thanks to Karen Goeltz, MD for helping with the ER section.

Notes

<u>Neurology</u>

For consultations: Why a neuro consult? What question needs to be answered?
Exam outline/briefing sequence:
        <u>Mental Status & Speech</u>
        CN (Cranial nerves)
        <u>Motor system</u>
        Coordination (cerebellum)
        <u>Sensory system</u>
        Pain, Temp
        Vibration
        Light touch
        Position
        Discriminative sensations
                Stereognosis
                Graphestesia
                2 point discrimination
                Point localization
                Extinction
        DTR (reflexes) & Babinski

Special
Aphasia
Asterixis
Winging Scapula
Meningeal signs
        Neck mobility
        Brudzinski's sign
        Kernig's sign

<u>Mental Status</u> (Alert & oriented to Person, Place & Time? Or...)
Is the patient on sedating meds? (i.e., midazolam, morphine, fentanyl, haldol, propofol) If so, ensure you note this.

Glasgow coma scale (3-15)

Eye opening	Motor response	Verbal response
	6 – obeys commands	
	5 – localizes to pain	5 - oriented
4 – spontaneous	4 – withdraws	4 - confused
3 – to sound	3 – flexion	3 - inappropriate
2 – to pain	2 – extension	2 - incomprehensible
1 – never	1 – none	1 - none

Ex. Pt is intubated & sedated on Versed 5 & Morphine 5 opens eyes to sound and localizes to pain (usually GCS # is used in the ER, on the floors spell it out in words).

close your eyes

Cognition (Mini mental Exam)
*Orientation:
  Person?
  (5) Place (country, state, city, hospital, floor)
  (5) Time (year, season, month, date, day of week)
*Registration:
  (3) Blue ball
       Red apple
       Yellow truck [pt repeats; tell pt to remember]
Attention&Calc:
  (5) count backwards by 7 or 3 [start at 100] (or spell 'world' backwards)
*Recall:
  (3) name the objects (from registration)
Language:
  (2) observe and name a watch & pen
  (1) repeat: "no ifs, ands, or buts"
  (3) "take this sheet of paper in your right hand, fold it, and put it on the floor."
  (1) pt reads & obeys "close your eyes"
  (1) pt writes a sentence
  (1) pt copies interlocking pentagon design

(pts) in brackets
(23<= dementia/cognitive disorder)

Cranial nerves
I Smell

II Visual Acuity, fields, ocular fundi
Pupillary responses: direct response & consensual (L & R) (CN2/3)
   PERRLA (Pupils Equal, Round, Reactive to Light & Accommodation)
Ophthalmoscope exam (pupillary responses 1st)
Visual acuity (L/R) (14" away; note glasses/contacts)
Visual fields (L/R) (test each eye, of quadrant separately)

CN III, IV, VI
Follow finger: 'H'
Convergence (arm's length to 6")
Near response (pt looks near, far; pupil changes)
Ptosis?

CN V$_1$, V$_2$, V$_3$
Motor: Feel masseter/temporal muscles (as pt bites down)
Sensory: sharp/dull - broken end of Q-tip (wooden)
         light touch - cotton ball (corneal reflex)

CN VII
Eyebrows, Frown, Show teeth, Smile, Puff out cheeks
Close eyes very tight - against resistance (L/R)

CN VIII
Whisper test (2ft) or finger rub (10cm)
Otoscope exam [tympanic membrane (perforation, inflammation, mobility, ossicles)]
         [external auditory meatus]
Rinne test (512 Hz) (L & R)
   place on mastoid process; 'tell me when you don't hear the sound'
   then, move in front of ear canal
         [conductive loss: Bone C.>Air C. or BC=AC]
         [sensorineural loss: AC>BC (which is normal)]
Weber test (512 Hz) (on skin, center of top of head)
         'where do you hear the sound?'
         [conductive loss: hear better in this ear]
         [sensorineural loss: can't hear in bad ear]

CN IX & X
Is voice nasal/hoarse? Difficult swallowing? Observe elev of palate "ah" (CN 10)
Gag reflex

CN XI
Rotate head against resistance (L & R), Shrug shoulders against resistance (L & R)

CN XII
Protrude tongue (directly out, move side to side), Strength of tongue (via cheek)

Motor system (Muscle strength)
Deltoid (push on abducted arms)
Biceps   (C5, 6)
Triceps   (C6, 7, 8)
Wrist (extend)
Grip (flex wrist&fingers)   (C7, 8, T1)
Fingers (extend)

Recumbent
Hip flexor   (L2, 3, 4) **(raise knee)**
Knee Flex
Knee Extend
Plantar flex foot   (S1) (**'push'**)
Dorsiflex foot   (L4, 5) (**'pull'**)

Coordination (cerebellum)
Romberg Test (stand, eyes closed for 15 sec) (look for sway)
Drift test (arms in front, eyes closed, and palms up, 15 sec)
Tap foot on floor (L/R)
Tap finger to thumb (L/R)
[Dysdiadochokinesis: if pt can't rapidly alt movements]
finger-to nose coord. (L/R)

Gait
walk away (observe gait & sensorium)
walk back on tip toes
walk away, on heels
walk back, heel-to-toe (like walking a line)

Sensory system (Pain, Temp, Vibration, Light touch, Position)
Vibration [128 HZ] Demo; Test (close eyes, each big toe or each ankle, pt states when vibration stops; pt>examiner)
Sharp vs. dull - broken end of Q-tip (wooden)
Light touch - cotton ball
Position: Toe/finger, show up/down, then eyes closed, test up vs. down - patient states 'up' or 'down'

Lower extremities (L/R)		Abdomen/Trunk (L/R)		Upper extremities (L/R)	
Lateral malleolus	(S1)	Arm pit level	(T2)	Clavicle	(C5)
Dorsum of foot	(L5)	Nipple	(T4)	Thumb	(C6)
Knee (outer)	(L5)	Xyphoid	(T6)	Index finger	(C7)
Medial malleolus	(L4)	Umbilicus	(T10)	little finger	(C8)
Big toe (outer)	(L4)	Iliac crest	(T12)		
Shin (below knee)	(L4)	Inguinal ligament	(L1)		
Knee (inner)	(L3)	Femoral pulse	(L2)		

Discrimitive sensation - cortex
Stereognosis - ability to identify an object by feeling it
Graphesthesia - write a number on the hand
[if can't perform these - lesion in sensory cortex]
Point localization
Extinction
2 point discrimination

DTR (reflexes)
       Biceps (palpate w/finger, strike)
       Brachioradialis (radius, 2" above wrist)
       Triceps
       Patellar
       Achilles
       Babinski
Special
Aphasia - disorder of comprehension or use of words or symbolic language arising from anatomical lesions in the dominant hemisphere.
Asterixis - "stop traffic"; hold arms out, with hands cocked up and fingers spread. Watch for 1-2 min. [sudden, brief, nonrhythmic flexion of the hands and fingers]
Winging of scapula - serratus anterior weakness or long thoracic nerve damage

Meningeal signs (Neck mobility)
Brudzinski's sign - (if no injury to the cervical vertebra, then chin to chest. [If pain then =>meningeal inflammation, arthritis, or neck injury; if hips and knees flex => + Brudzinski's sign]
Kernig's sign - supine; flex hip to 90°; straighten the knee [pain (not discomfort) and increased resistance is + Kernig's sign; if bilateral then Meningeal irritation]
Anal reflex - using a dull object, stroke outward in the 4 quadrants from the anus; there should be a reflexive contraction of the anus musculature [loss of the anal reflex suggests a lesion in S2-4 reflex arc - a cauda equina lesion]

Comatose patient
Alertness - speaking normally, an alert patient opens eyes, looks at you, and responds fully.
Lethargy - speak in a loud voice [appears drowsy but opens eyes, answers questions, and goes back to sleep]
Obtundation - shake the pt gently [opens eyes, looks at you confused and responds slowly]
Stupor   - apply a painful stimulus (pinch a tendon, rub the sternum, roll a pencil across the nailbed) [stuporous patient arouses from sleep, slow verbal responses, goes back into an unresponsive state without the pain]
Coma   - apply repeated painful stimuli [eyes closed, no evidence of response]

References: Bickley, LS. Bates' Guide to Physical Examination and History Taking, 7th edition, Lippincott Williams & Wilkins, Philadelphia, 1999.

Notes

Pediatrics

<u>Child History</u>
Name, Age, Sex, Birthdate
Address   **Telephone #**
Informant (reliability)
Date and Time of admission

Chief Complaints (CC): Patient's/Parent's: why at the hospital (w/ duration)

History of Present Illness: times (relative to admission); chronological
  Onset, Location, Duration, Quality, Intensity, Radiation, Exacerbation,
  Alleviation, Setting it occurs, Assoc. symptoms, Past hist, Freq
  [Pertinent (-); pull up into HPI pertinent info., ER presentation]
  [interventions made & admission rsn; ddx should be apparent based on Qs]
  Current Medications: dose & freq. (any pill/herb)

Past History:
  Prev. Illnesses/infections: experienced or recent exposure to (MMR,
    whoop cough, chicken pox, rheumatic & scarlet F, polio)
  Hospitalizations: hosp, Dx, Rx, length
  Injuries: nature, complications
  Operations: hosp, type of operation, complications
  Immunizations: number, dates (HBV, DPT, OPV, MMR, Hib, PPD)
  Allergies (meds, eczema, urticaria, rhinitis, asthma, food, insect) w/specific rxn

Perinatal Hist: (if<2 or neuro/develop problems)
 Prenatal: preg order, mom's health, clinic visits, serology, blood type, illnesses (Fever, rashes), medications, bleeding; -OH, smoke, drugs
 Natal: duration of preg., location, duration of labor, presentation, delivery (method, sedation, anesthesia), length of hosp.
 Postnatal: gen condition, 1st cry, respirations (spontaneous onset time or resuscitation); Complications (convulsions, rash, hemorrhage, jaundice, resp. distress, cyanosis, anemia, congen. anomalies, infection), feedings, duration of hosp stay, birth wt, length & head circumference. APGAR score; gestational age; Patterns (crying, sleeping, urination, defecation)

Nutrition History: (if<2)
  Infancy: feeding method (breast, formula type, combo), qty and freq (for 24hrs) duration, time of intro of (solid foods, vitamins (type, dose), water source) feeding difficulties (appetite, allergy), wt gain, current diet & nutrition
  Childhood: Eating habits (likes/dislikes), typical types and amounts, parental ideas about eating, body perceptions

Growth & Development History
  [Physical growth- growth chart]
  Age of: head control, smile, grasp and transfer, roll over, crawl, sit, walk unassisted, talk (1st word, 2 word & 3 word sentences), toilet training and age approp. milestones (DDST – current milestones), grade in school and school performance

[Health Maintenance]
Immunizations
Screenings (BP, vision, hearing, TB, blood levels, urinalysis, PKU,
galactosemia, HbSS, alpha-1-anti-trp)
Safety & Injury prevention ('anticipatory guidance to Mom & Dad')
<u>**General**</u>
Sleep on back (prevent SIDS)
Car seat (+2 =>face front)
Seat belt=> if +4yr or 40lbs
If guns =>lock them up
Smoking/fire detector/burns (water)
Brother/Sister? =>sicknesses
Honey=>Bot tox
TV vs. reading & physical fitness (play)
Nutrition (no solids until 4-6 mo)
Discipline (appropriate for age-parents)
Poisoning; Falls; Drowning
Toys (safe for age)
Park – strangers
Sleep schedule

<u>**Age: 3-4-5: separation issues (to preschool)**</u>
Know 1st and last name, address, phone #
Strangers & If anyone touches private parts tell mommy
Practice getting up early, 1mo before
Practice deciding about cloths
Parents: ask what happened during the day
Family dinner – together is important

<u>**Adolescents**</u>
Sex/ SDTs/ Drugs/Alcohol/smoking
Risky behavior/ fights/ School performance
Hygiene

Family History: age, health & Illnesses
   Parents: ages, race, occupation, state of health
   Siblings: chrono order, sex, state of health
   Diseases: (HbSS, DM, hyperlipidemia, cardio, HTN, cancer, etc.),
      family history of child's problem?

Social & Environmental History: Family home; apt vs. house, urban vs. rural;
   # people in house; $ support and health coverage

Personal History: Sleep & eat habits; urinary & bowel control;
   disturbances (bed wetting, thumb sucking, temper tantrums,
   abnormal ties to parents), relation with peers

28

Review of Systems (ROS):
General: change of weight, pattern of growth, fatigue/ weakness, onset of puberty, fever/ chills/ sweats
Neuromuscular: headache, dizziness, ataxia, convulsions
Skin & Mucous membranes: pallor, jaundice, rashes, epistaxis, abscesses
Respiratory: colds (description, #/yr), sore throats, otitis media, pneumonia, wheezing
Cardiovascular: dyspnea, cyanosis, hear murmurs, syncope, orthopnea, "blue baby"
Gastrointestinal: appetite, nausea, vomiting, abd. pains, diarrhea, constipation, encopresis
Genitourinary: infections, frequency, dysuria, nocturia, hematuria, urgency, dribbling, enuresis, oliguria, force of stream
Extremities: joint pains, fractures, limping, deformities

Old Charts:
Summarize

Physical Exam
Temp (oral/rectal), BP (arm/leg, L/R), Pulse, RR,
Body measurements & %iles (wt, length, height & head circumference)
General Inspection: ill/well; acute/chronic; distress, alert, cooperative, body build, nutrition, hydration, dysmorphic features, behavior.
Skin: color (pale, cyanotic, jaundice), eruption (papular, macular, vesicular) hemorrhagic manifestations and location, turgor, edema.
Head: size, shape, fontanelles (size, tension, closed/open), sutures, scalp hair
Eye: ptosis, strabismus, conjunctivae, sclerae, pupils, extraocular muscles, fundus (vessels, hemorrhage, disc), red reflex
Nose: discharge, flaring of alae nasi, airway obstruction
Mouth & throat: lips, tooth (#, caries), mucosa (color, enanthem, dry or moist)
tongue, gum, palate, uvula, pharynx (injection), tonsils (size, injection, exudates)
Neck: position (tort Collis, tilting, mobility), lymph nodes, stiffness, masses, SCMs, trachea, thyroid.
Chest: shape, rosary, expansion, retraction, & symmetry; chest wall masses or tenderness.
Lungs: inspection (rate, type, depth, dyspnea), palpation (fremitus), percussion (dullness, resonance), auscultation (fine or coarse rales, rhonchi, wheezes).
Heart: inspection (precordial bulge, impulse, clubbing), palpation (apex impulse, thrill), auscultation (sounds, rhythm, quality, split, third sound, friction rub, murmur – describe nature), peripheral pulses.
Abdomen: size & contour, visible peristalsis, veins, umbilicus, tenderness, rebound tenderness & rigidity, shifting dullness, palpable organs or masses, bowel sounds (hyperactive, normoactive, hypoactive).
Genitalia: male – (phimosis, testes, hernia, hydrocele, penile discharge, circumcised)
Female – (labia, vagina, clitoris, hernia, vaginal discharge)
Rectum & anal margin: findings on rectal examination if done; tone of external anal sphincter, anal fissures.
Extremities: anomalies, deformity, posture, joints (if abnormal inspection, movement, palpation, and measurement), edema; hand and feet, nails (clubbing, cyanosis).
Lymph nodes: occipital, cervical, axillary, inguinal, size, redness, consistency, mobility, tenderness.
Nervous system: cerebral function (level of consciousness, orientation, etc.), CN, cerebellar function (coordination, tremor, ataxia, etc.), motor system (muscle strength, spontaneous movement, involuntary movement, gait), reflexes (deep tendon, superficial, pathological Kernig, Brudzinski, primitive reflexes).

29

<u>Lab Values</u>
Problem list
Provisional diagnosis
ddx: (in order of likelihood w/reasonable discussion)
Diagnostic plan: (tests)
Therapeutic plan: (meds)

<u>PE (<1yr)</u>
Feel fontanelles
Ear psn
Inspect face
Suck finger/feel palate
Look for symmetrical movements
Feel for grasp reflex bilaterally & try to lift own wt.
Lymph nodes
Clavicles feel
Red reflex – eyes
EOMI?
Heart
Abdomen
Femoral & radial pulses
Check hips for clicks
Foot grasp
Moro reflex (2-4 mo it's lost)-symmetry

APGAR scoring exam:
<u>Appearance</u>
2 Entire body pink
1 Pink body with blue extremities
0 Entire body blue or pale
<u>Pulse</u>
2 >100 beats/min
1 <100 beats/min
0 absent
<u>Grimace</u>
2 Cough, sneeze, or vigorous cry
1 Grimace or slight cry
0 No response
<u>Activity</u>
2 Active movement
1 Some movement
0 Limp, motionless
<u>Respirations</u>
2 Strong, crying
1 Slow, irregular
0 Absent

30

Breast Feeding/Nutritional requirements

How do you know an infant is hungry? (**Crying does not always mean hunger**)
- Infants that awaken and cry at short intervals might not receive enough @ feeding
- Crying can be caused by: hunger, too much clothing, colic, soiled/wet/uncomfortable diapers, gas, too hot/ too cold, illness (Sick infants are not interested in food), a need to be held (if crying stops after being picked usu they do not need food)
-Still crying, after being held & offered food => search for other causes
Note: inconsolable crying = life threatening problem = get to the emergency room fast.

Breastfeeding vs. formula
Breast milk: the natural food for full-term infants during the first months of life:
- always available, proper temperature, no prep time, free of contaminating bacteria
- superior to formula for normal infants

	Human milk	Similac
kcal/oz	22	20
Protein	1.1	1.5
Carbohydrates	7.0	6.8
Fat	3.8	3.8
Na	6.5	7.0
K	14	14.7

Age	# feedings q24h
Birth - 1 wk	6-10
1 wk - 1 mo	6-8
1-3 mo	5-6
3-7 mo	4-5
4-9 mo	3-4
8-12 mo	3

Age	Qty @ each feeding
1-2 wk	2-3oz (60-90ml)
3 wk – 2 mo	4-5oz (120-150ml)
2 – 3 mo	5-6oz (150-180ml)
3 – 4 mo	6-7oz (180-210ml)
5 – 12 mo	7-8oz (210-240ml)

Note: 24hr feedings for 1-2 months; small/weak infants feed q2h-q3h; infants usu self regulate the quantity, but sufficient qty has to be offered.

Weaning (at 6-12mo infants)
- reduce volume and freq of milk; increase foods & liquids by bottle and cup
- the transition should be gradual, without conflict

Reference:
-H&P + ROS adapted from Jay Mayefsky, M.D., Department of Pediatrics, Cook County Hospital, Chicago, IL
-Nelson Textbook of Pediatrics, 16th Ed.

Notes

Psychiatry

History
CC
HPI
Past history (antecedents of Ψ disorder: gestation, birth, develop, head trauma, SZ, Xrays/MRI of your head, high fevers, viruses, street drugs)
Past Ψ history
Family history
Social history
Behavioral Exam

Behavioral Exam
Appearance:
Body type: (endomorphic-chubby, ecto-thin, meso-avg), age, ethnicity, sex
Alertness: alert, drowsy, stupor, comatose, (A&O x 4 = person, place, time, & situation)
Attentiveness: attentive, disinterested, bored, internally preoccupied, distractible
Cooperativeness: cooperative, guarded, suspicious
Dress: fashionable, well fitting, well matched, unstained
Grooming: hygiene, unkept
Distinguishing Features: Scars, needle pucture wounds, tattoos, bandages, bloodstains, missing teeth, tobacco-stained fingers
Physical abnormalities: missing limbs, pallor, cyanosis, jaundice, profuse sweating, goiter, wheezing, coughing
Emotional facial expressioning: sitting calmly, crying, omega sign (furrowed brow), looking as if listening to voices

Global Motor Function:
Activity: hyper, hypoactivity, agitation (↑motor) (pacing, fidgety, unable to sit still, wringing hands, rocking), bradykinesia (↓motor)
Abnormal movements: tremor (resting/intention), dyskinesia (abnormal movements) lip smacking, tongue thrusts, mannerisms, tics, apraxia (not able to perform simple motor tasks despite normal strength)
Gait: normal, shuffling, broad based, stumbling, limping
Catatonia: stupor w/mutism (akinetic mutism), excitement, waxy flexibility, stereotypy (repeated movements), verbigeration (repetition of words that are meaningless), palilalia (phrases are repeated freq w/inc rapidity), automatic obedience (pt responds to touch despite verbal commands), catalepsy (maintaining a psn for a while), echolalia/echopraxia (echo examiner's speech/movements)

Affect (Emotional Expression)
Mood range: constricted, full, increased, decreased
Intensity: flat, blunted, exaggerated
Quality: sad, irritable, elated, apprehension, euphoric, apathetic, depressed, happy, angry, anxious
Affect/mood: stable, fixed, labile
Appropriateness: to content of speech circumstances
Relatedness: (with me during conversation; able to convey one's feelings empathically to others)
Facial expressions/hand gestures:
Volition: ideas, plans, interests, activities, concerns for the present and future
Emotional blunting: loss of emotional expression & avolition

Speech & Language: (Articulation: clear, mumbled, slurred, dysarthric)
Turn taking: Intrusive w/press of speech [M,drug]; Paucity [D, drug, post-ictal, motor aphasia, L basal ganglia, thalamic]
Fluency: reduced (few words) [D, S, motor aphasia]; reduced & halting [broca, ictal]; increased (too many words) [M, drug, anxiety]
Distractibility: increased (jump topic to topic) [M, drug, delirium, anxiety]; decreased [melancholia]
Spontaneity: Overly [M, drug]; reduced [D, S, post-ictal, drug, metabolic, Broca/motor aphasia, L basal ganglia & thalamic]
Organization (syntax/word usage/logic): disorganized w/paraphasias [S, Hallucinations, drug psychosis, SZ of dominant front-temp, thalamic, aphasia]

Types of Aphasias	Spontaneous	Fluency	comprehension	repetition	organization
Broca's:	dysarthric	not	reduced	labored/telegraphic	telegraphic
Transcortical motor:	dysarthric	not	ok	can repeat some	paucity/org ok/diff reading aloud
Transcortical sensory: naming,reading,writing	normal	fluent	poor	normal	paraphasic/poor
Wernicke's: naming,reading,writing	normal	fluent	poor	poor	paraphasic/poor

Thought Process:
Non-Formal Thought Disorder: flight of ideas [M], circumstantial (does answer the question) [M, aging, epilepsy, drug users], rambling speech
FTD: aphasic, nonsequiturs (pt's response is unrelated to question), tangentially (doesn't reach point), word approximations ('writer' for pen), private word usage, neologisms (new words are meaningless), perseveration (repetition of stock words, just added into speech), verbigeration (repeating associations, esp. at the end of sentences), driveling (jargon-unfamiliar language), derailment, thought blocking, word salad, elliptical speech

Thought Content:
Suicidal/Homicidal ideation, assaultive
1st Rank Sx[S]: 1. CAH complete auditory hallucination (voice heard and sustained)
2. Exp. of control (outside force controls thoughts, feelings, or actions)
3. Experience of alienations (actions are someone else's)
4. Thought broadcasting (other people can hear Pt's thoughts)
5. Delusional perception (giving delusions meaning to real objects)
Delusions (fixed false beliefs): of perception (a real perception is personalized), systematic(details like a movie plot), grandiose, persecutory, of guilt, ideas of

34

reference(people's actions relate to you), of influence, organized/disorganized, mood congruent(e.g., being persecuted for bad things done), nihilistic (thinks oneself does not exist), overvalued ideas (a person's energy is all related to one idea), 1°/2° delusion (delusion due to the 1° delusion)

Perceptual: other hallucinations (auditory, visual, olfactory, gustatory, tactile)(perceptions without external stimuli), illusions (misinterpretation of sensory information), elementary/complex, dysmorphopsia (changes in object shape), micro/macro/dysmegalopsia (changes in object size), hyper/hypoacusia (distortion of sound perception), extracampine (outside normal sensory field; i.e. hear people talking in other rooms), dejavu/jamais vu (the illusion that something has already been experienced or seen/never experienced despite it being familiar [temporal lesion]), depersonalization, derealization.

Cognition (5 stages)
1. **Global Assessment:** responds to questions; focus attention on examiner; not distracted; doesn't doze
2. **Attention/Concentration:** 'A' test
3. **Speech and Language:** (above)
4. **Screening:** MMSE (30)
[<22 demented; 23-26 2° behavioral conditon;27-30 severe 1° behavioral syn/elderly]
5. **Additional testing: (optional)**

Motor signs: (L/R, front/back, top/bottom)
  Front/Top:Frontal lobe: impersistence, preservation, inertia, overflow sequencing, perseveration, dysarthria
  Front/Bottom:Basal Ganglia: [mood, motor, memory] resting tremor, choreiform mvnmts (motor overflow), bradykinesia, flexed posture, inc muscle tone/floppy
  Back:Cerebellar/Pons: intentional tremors, past pointing, dysmetria, dysdiadochokinesia (not able to rapidly alt movements), poor (ataxia, tandem gait), Romberg sign
  Top:Parietal lobe: (kinesthetic, spatial neglect, stereoagnosia, graphesthesis, constructional/dressing ideomotor apraxia, calculating, writing, reading aloud, Anosognosia (awareness of disease)
  Temporal: receptive language, memory
Judgement: problem solving skills
Memory - immediate, recent, remote, constructional abilities

<u>Screening Questions</u> **Was there ever a time when... (if + go to more detailed qstns)**
Depression: you felt down in the dumps, blue, depressed for days/weeks?
Mania: for days or weeks you had unusual amounts of energy/full of ideas/ did a lot/ talked a lot/felt really happy or emotional?
Volition: What do you do to keep busy? For fun? Hobbies or interests?
Perceptual Disturbances: Has anything strange happened to your hearing of vision?
Delusions: Have you ever felt that someone was: spying on you? Following you? Plotting against you? Trying to harm you?
Alcohol Screening: (CAGE) Ever felt the need to cut down? Annoyed by criticism? Guilty about drinking? Ever drink in the morning (eye opener)?
Street Drugs: Have you ever used street drugs?
Anxiety disorder: Are you a nervous person? Ever suddenly feel your heart pounding for no apparent reason? (Tight chest? SOB? Breathing fast? Feel your heart beating? Pins & needles in your hands/feet/lips? Headaches or dizzy?)

Assessment & Plan
  Axis I: Clinical disorders
  Axis II: Personality disorders, mental retardation
 Axis III: General medical conditions
 Axis IV: Ψ social and enviro problems (stressful events relevant to mental disorder)
  Axis V: Global Assessment of Functioning (GAF) (Clinician's judgment of
Individual's overall level of functioning; 100=no Sx, 50=some persistent
  danger to self/others;<35=hospitalization)

Detailed Screening Questions

Depression
1. Have you ever felt down, depressed for days/weeks without anything cheering you up (such as friends/family/the things you enjoy)?
2. Did it affect you're appetite or sleep? Tell me about your sleep.
3. When you were depressed:
        Did you worry?
        Could you concentrate?
        Did you want to go to sleep and never wake up?
        Did you want to die?
        Did you think about harming yourself?
        Lose interest in hobbies, work, and sex?
        Did it keep you from doing things?

Mania
1. Have you ever had unusual amounts of energy where you were full of ideas, did a lot, talked a lot for days or weeks? Too emotional, too happy, to hyper, too high?
2. Have you ever had racing thoughts or a lot of ideas? Trouble concentrating? Trouble sitting still? Always seem to be on the go? Have big plans? Have special abilities or powers ordinary people do not have?

Emotional Blunting (things to notice)
1. Prosody (rhythm, melody or articulation of speech): Facial expression, tone of voice, gestures, eye contact.
2. Volition: What do you to keep busy? Fun activities (hobbies)? Do you have friends or family? What are your future plans? Do you mind being in the hospital? If you had to stay 2 months how would you feel?

Perceptual Disturbances
Have you been hearing unusual, odd or strange noises/voices? Is someone talking to you, commenting on things you're doing? Do you hear people talking about you?

Delusions
Have you ever felt that someone was: spying on you? Plotting against you? Trying to harm you? Do you think you are a special person, or have special talents or powers ordinary people do not have?

Alcohol Screening
1. Some people who get some relief from alcohol. How about you?
    a. Do you use alcohol?
    b. Has anyone ever though you were drinking too much?
    c. How much do you drink each day?
    d. Do you get shakes from stopping suddenly? Longest time without a drink?
    e. Any blackouts? Any DUIs, disorderly conduct?
    f. Have you ever tried to stop? Ever drink in the morning?

Street Drugs
Have you ever used street drugs? If yes…What happened?

Anxiety disorder
1. Are you a nervous person?
2. Do you get nervous in elevators, around heights, animals, around lots of people, travel away from home, around new people?
3. Ever feel your heart racing for no apparent reason? When it happens, do you have:
    a. Tight chest? SOB? Breathing fast?
    b. Pins & needles in your hands/feet/lips? Headaches or dizzy?
4. Do you spend a lot of time checking things you have already done?
    a. How many times do you check?
    b. Do your family/friends complain about this?
    c. Do you think you do it too much?
5. Some people are concerned about germs; always washing. Are you like that?
6. Have you ever had something frightening happen to you, and then for weeks/months after you were nervous and you kept on re-living it? Did it affect your work, or personal life?

Preexisting conditions
1. Did your mother have a difficult pregnancy with you? Was she ever concerned about your health, as a baby, as a result?
    a. Did you have difficult walking/talking or doing anything? Were you healthy?
    b. Did you ever have any serious medical conditions?
2. Have you ever lost consciousness? How long? Did you have to stay overnight at a hospital? Did it affect you're: vision, concentration, balance, memory, headaches?
3. Have you ever had seizures? EEG? X-rays of your head?

4. Have you ever experienced:
   a. Sudden changes in: vision, hearing, taste, smell, feelings in your body?
   b. You went to a familiar place but didn't recognize it?
   c. You went to an unfamiliar place, but it seemed as if you had been there before?
   d. Everyday objects seemed to change in size or shape right in from of your eyes?

Frontal Lobe testing
[dysfunction: if Broca's/transcortical motor aphasia; avolition; loss of emotional expression [ND]; catatonia; frontal/basal ganglia motor signs; obsessive-compulsive; poor judgment (daily living: impulsivity, can't see one's shortcomings, unrealistic plans); inappropriate social behaviors (intrusive/unkept/dirty); perseveration
Testing:
1. Generation of ideas: 1min – name as many animals as possible (>15 normal)
2. Problem solving: 18 books, 2 shelves, 2x top as bottom, how many on each shelf? (T12/B6)
3. Thinking: how are items similar? [airplane/bike; desk/chair]

Dementia testing
Digit span: [attention, concentration, & immediate auditory memory]
1. Sensitive to general deterioration of the brain (early Alzheimer's)
2. Examiner says sequence and pt repeats back (forward, then backward #)
3. Scores: add highest # forward to highest # in reverse.
   a. low=anxiety, major depression w/psychotic features
   b. L hemisphere: uses digits fwd & back
   c. R hemisphere uses digits backward
4. rules: two tries at each length, if miss, then stop
5. Normal Score: a. 16yr: 14 b. 50yr: 15; c. 70yr: 13

Digits forward (max 9) + **Digits backward** (max 8) = max 17

5-8-2	6-9-4
6-4-3-9	7-2-8-6
4-2-7-3-1	7-5-8-3-6
6-1-9-4-7-3	3-9-2-4-8-7
5-9-1-7-4-2-8	4-1-7-9-3-8-6
5-8-1-9-2-6-4-7	3-8-2-9-5-1-7-4
2-7-5-8-6-2-5-8-4	

Mini Mental Exam (used as a screening tool)

Close your eyes

<u>Cognition</u>
*Orientation:
Person?
(5) Place (country, state, city, hospital, floor)
(5) Time (year, season, month, date, day of week)
*Registration:
(3) Blue ball
Red apple
Yellow truck [pt repeats; tell pt to remember]
Attention&Calc:
(5) count backwards by 7 or 3 [start at 100] (or spell 'world' backwards)
*Recall:
(3) name the objects (from registration)
Language:
(2) observe and name a watch & pen
(1) repeat: "no ifs, ands, or buts"
(3) "take this sheet of paper in your right hand, fold it, and put it on the floor."
(1) pt reads & obeys "close your eyes"
(1) pt writes a sentence
(1) pt copies interlocking pentagon design

(pts) in brackets
(23<= dementia/cognitive disorder)

M-mania D-depression S-schizophrenia SZ-seizure DM-dominant ND-nondominant

Reference
Adapted from the Chicago Medical School Clinical Neuroscience/ Psychiatry Course

Notes

Obstetrics & Gynecology

OB/GYN H&P (usually there is a form to fill out)

Date: Time:
Age: Gravida: # Para: # # # #   FDLMP: EDC:
                                        PMP: GA:
CC/HPI/ROS:
(FM) Fetal movements? (LOF) leakage of fluid? (VB) Vaginal bleeding? Pain? (CTX)
contractions? Burning with urination? Frequency (urine)? (HA) Headache? Blurred
vision/visual changes? (RUQ) Right Upper Quadrant Pain? Edema?

Prenatal Physician:

Prenatal care:
Date of first visit: How far pregnant (at first visit):
Ultrasounds(dates):
Special procedures:

LABS:
PAP Smear: (date & +/-)   MSAFP:
H/H: # / #   Blood Group: (Ab+/Ab-)   Sickling: (+/-)
Rubella: immune? RPR: NR?   VDRL: (+/-)   PPD: (+/-)
HbSAg: (+/-)   Hep C: (+/-)   Hep A: (+/-)   PLT: #
GBS: (+/-)   GC: (+/-)   Chlamydia: (+/-)   HSV: (+/-)

Medications: (current and during pregnancy)
Allergies:
Labs:

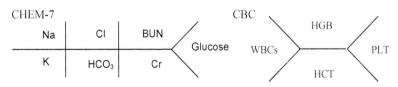

Albumin:
Total Protein:
Uric Acid:
ALT:
AST:
ALP:

UA: Protein:

History

Births:

Name	DOB/yr	Route	Weight	M/F	complications	hospital

Child #1
Child #2
Child #3
(Route – NSVD or C/S (Why C/S?); Complications – i.e. cord, placenta, etc.)

PSH: previous surgeries
PMH: DM?, HTN?, etc.
SH: Smoking: ____PPD for ____yrs
        Alcohol:
        Drugs:
OB/GYN: Menarche Age:
         Birth control type:
         Operations: i.e. fibroid removal, etc.
         Infections: STDs
         Last Pap smear:
FH: Mom:
        Dad:
        Siblings:

Physical Exam

Date & Time:
Vitals: BP: T: P: RR:
General: Mental Status: HT: WT:
HEENT: (PEARRL, - Thyromegaly, etc.)
CV: (S1S2, RRR, - Murmur, etc.)
Pulm: (CTA, - rales, - rhonchi, etc.)
Breast:
Abd:
        Condition: EPWT:
        McDonald: #cm   FHT:
        Presentation: Toco:
Pelvic:
        Vulva:
        Vagina:
        Cervix: Dilatation: Effacement:
                Station: Position:
                BOW:
Ext: +/- Edema   DTRs:

Impression: 23yo G2P1001 IUP@ 31 3/7 wks admitted for preterm CTX. R/O pre-eclampsia.

Plan:

Definitions for H&P   GxPxxxx (Gravida/Para)

Gravida: # times preg with child

Para: 1. term live births (a viable infant [>500g or >20 weeks] regardless of whether the infant is alive at birth 2. spontaneous abortion 3. induced termination 4. # living children

FDLMP: first day of last menstrual period

EDC: est. date of confinement (est. delivery date)

PMP: previous menstrual period (the period before the LMP)

GA: gestational age

MSAFP: maternal serum alpha fetal protein

H/H: HGB/HCT

Ab: antibody

RPR: syphilis test (reactive or nonreactive)

VDRL: syphilis test (+ or -)

PPD: TB test (+/-)

HbSAg: Hepatitis surface antigen (+/-)

Hep C: Hepatitis C(+/-)

Hep A: Hepatitis A(+/-)

PLT: platelets (HELLP syn: severe pre-eclampsia characterized by: hemolysis, elevated liver enzymes, low platelets)

GBS: Group B Streptococcus infection (+/-)

GC: Gonococcus infection (Neisseria gonorrhoeae) (+/-)

HSV: Herpes Simplex Virus (+/-)

NSVD: normal spontaneous vaginal delivery

C/S: caesarian section

Condition: condition of the abdomen (gravid, NT, etc.)

EPWT: est. fetal weight (by US) (by leipold)

McDonald: distance in cm from pubic symphsis to top of fundus

Presentation: vertex – baby's head direction (by US) (by exam)

FHT: Fetal heart beat

Toco: contractions (Q 4-5min, etc.)

Vulva: with in normal limits?

Vagina: with in normal limits?

Cervix Dilatation: # cm

Cervix Effacement: %

Fetal Station: (i.e., -2, +2)

Fetal Position: (i.e., anterior, posterior)

BOW: Bag of water: (i.e. intact, ruptured, + nitrozine, + pooling, AFI #)

Fetal Heart Monitor

Look at 3 things:

1. **Baseline heart rate**: normal limits 110-160

2. **Variation**, from base line: should be at least 3-5 cycles (up and downward movement of the heart rate, from base line q min) (flat is bad; a jagged baseline is good)

3. **Reactivity**: Reactive if: there are 2 accelerations q 20min (each acceleration must be 15sec long and 15bpm above baseline)

Decelerations (FHM +Toco)
1. **Early**: if the decal starts and ends with contractions [fetal head compressed causes ↑ vagal tone and ↓ HR]
2. **Variable**: usu drop fast [umbilical cord compression, repeated in series: cord entrapped under shoulder/around neck
3. **Late**: start at the peak of the contraction (usu uteroplacental insufficiency – most worrisome)

Amniotic Membrane Rupture Proof
+ Nitrazine, + fluid in vaginal vault, + Ferning, AFI (amniotic fluid index – US)

Obstetric SOAP note
S: Fetal movements? Contractions? Leakage of fluid? R upper Quadrant pain? Vaginal bleeding? Pain? Pre-eclamptic: (SOB? HA? Blurred vision? Dizzy? Swelling of hands and face?)
O: last 3 BP readings　　　　P　　　　RR
General: Mental Status
CV:
Pulm:
FHT: fetal heart tones
TOCO: contractions
SVE: sterile vaginal exam

Pre-eclamptic pts also:
Abd: RUQ:
Ext:　　　DTR: (hyper Mg = hyporeflexia)
spO_2

Labs
Pre-eclamptic pts: LFTS, Uric acid, BUN, Cr
I/O:

A/P: Age G#P# @ # wks IUP...
(Pitocin? Mg? Foley bulb? Expectant management? Dexamethasone? UTI – Abx? GBS+ PCN? Chorioamnioitis? etc.)

GYN Post Op Notes
S: how does the pt feel? bleeding? Pain? N/V? Bowel movement/flatus? SOB? Chest pain? Ambulation (after 6-8hrs)? Spirometer being used (prevents atelectasis #1 cause of fever)? Staple removal 7-10 days.
O: Vitals: Tmax　　BP　　　P　　　RR
MS: alert & Ox3?
CV:
Pulm:
Abd: BS? NT? distended? incision: erythema? bleeding? tenderness? (look under dressing after 48 hrs), dehiscence?
Ext: edema? Homan's sign (dorsiflex foot & squeeze calf gently, if pain= +)?
I/O
Meds:
Labs: CBC, BMP
A/P: # yo POD #1 s/p procedure...

44

Post Partum SOAP
NSVD

S: how does the pt feel? Vaginal bleeding? Pain? Headache? Blurred vision? Bowel movement/flatus? How does pt plan on feeding baby (breast/bottle)? Plan for contraception? Depression?

O: Vitals: Tmax   BP   P   RR
CV:
Pulm:
Abd: RUQ pain? Fundal height and firmness (usu. firm and below umbilicus)?
Ext: edema? Homan's sign (dorsiflex foot & squeeze calf gently, if pain= +)?

Labs:
H/H
GBS (if + pt usu stays 2 days)
RPR (if reactive, Penicillin G and 3 day stay)
HIV (if + no breast feeding)
Rubella
Hep B (if + and LFTs↑ then no breast feeding)
GC
Chlamydia
Type and screen

A/P: 25 yo G3P3 s/p NSVD @ 39wk IUP, delivered 3/14/04 at 1500hrs. Pt doing well, plan discharge home.

C/S (additional things)
-Fluids: I/O oligouric? Normal urine output 30cc/hr.
-Incisions: check @ 24-48hrs; erythema, pus, bleeding?
-Spirometer: ensure pt is using (atelectasis is #1 cause for fever in 1st 24hrs)
-Complications:
  • Bleeding (hypotension, tachycardia, abd distention)
  • MI: chest pain, dyspnea
  • PE: occurs in 1:5000 post partum pts: dyspnea, chest pain (oral contraceptive pills ↑ risk for PE, therefore wait 6 weeks)
-Can walk usually in 6-8 hours
-Staples removed: 7-10days
-RTC if Fever
    0-24 hrs: Atelectasis, chorioamnionitis
    24-48 hrs: UTI
-C/S pts usually stay 2-3 days

Discharge Plans (usually)
Motrin 600mg PO Q4-6hr prn for pain (x 1-2 months)
FeSO$_4$ 325mg QD if HGB (10-12), BID if HGB (8-10), TID if HGB (<8) (x 1month)
Colace 100mg PO BID (x 1-2 months)
Diet: regular
Instructions: no sex, no tampons, no douching for 6 wks, RTC 6 wks
Reference:
H&P adapted from the Mt. Sinai hospital H&P form, Chicago, IL
Other information obtained via personal experience on the OB/GYN rotation

Notes

Templates

Admission Orders/Post operative orders:
Admit to: floor c telemetry   **Service:**   **Attending:**
Diagnosis/procedure:
Condition:
Vitals [Q1/2/4/6, routine, neuro/vasc checks]
Activity [bed rest, ad lib, OOB to chair, ambulate TID
Diet [NPO (hold DM meds/slide scale), clears, regular, ADA]
I/Os [strict, routine]
IVF [Hep-lock IV, NS or LR(Cr)]
    PRBC, FFP, Cryoprecipitate, Platelets
Nursing
    Weights [now, daily weights]
    Drains (record drain output q shift)
        NGT to low intermittent or low constant (if sump)(flush NGT 30 ccNS Qshift)
        Penrose
        JP to bulb suction
        foley to gravity
        chest tube to -20 water suction
    DVT: [SCDs while in bed, Heparin 5000U SQ BID, lovenox]
    Glucose checks (Q6h, QAC&HS)
Meds
    Gtts/drips/pressors
    O2
    Pain (Narcotics +/- Tylenol)
    Antibiotics
    Protonix
    Steroids Hydrocortisone 100mg IVQ8h, Taper, Synthroid
    Cardiac (Digoxin, B Blocker; Not ACE/Ca blocker post op)
    DM: (not oral, slide scale, gluc check Q6h, call if >150)
    Anticoagulation: Heparin/Coumadin/ (lovenox not true anticoag)
    Drug levels
    Alcohol withdrawal [benzos, vit B]
    Nausea [Zofran, Phenergan, Tigan]
    Sleepers [Benadryl, zoloft]
Allergies
Labs [Now, tonight, in am](Nephro panel+Mg, CBC, coags, LFTSs, ABG)
Monitors [telemetry, BP cuff, CVP, Central, Swann, a-line]
Respiratory care [ISB 2 puff Q10min while awake, Bipap 5/10, EZPAP, Albuterol/Atrovent nebs Q4]
Vent settings [ABG 1h, pCXR]
Dressing Care [W→D BID c dakins]
Consults [PT/OT/Social services]
HO Call [T>38.5, spO2% <90%, P>100 or <60, SBP>160 or <100, RR>20, MS changes, UO<60 ml over 2h]
Pacemaker interrogation
Preop [NPO-IVF, Nephro panel+Mg, CBCcdiff, coags, UA+C&S, EKG, CXR, T&S/C, abx, GI preps, consent, anesthesia]

Admit orders: Remember "ADC VANDALISM"
1) Admit: floor, room, team, attending, residents
2) Diagnosis: list in order of priority
3) Condition: good, stable, fair, guarded, critical, etc.
4) Vitals: q4hrs, q shift, routine, etc.
5) Allergies
6) Nursing orders: call physician if...BP↓, RR, PR, Temp, UO
        SCDs, Foley, incentive spirometry, dressing care
7) Diet: regular, ADA (diabetic), low sodium, clear liquid, NPO, etc.
8) Activity: as tolerated, bed rest, up to chair, ambulate with assist, Full, etc.
9) Labs: CBC, BMP, Liver profile and when to draw.
10) Ins and Outs: strict, routine, ad lib, etc.
        IV fluids: D%NS to run at 120 ml/hr, etc.
        Drains: Foley to gravity, NGT to intermittent suction, etc.
11) Special orders: pCXR, EKG
12) Meds: insulin, pain meds, DVT prophylaxis, abx, etc.
13) Monitors: arterial line, noninvasive BP, CVP, pulse ox.

SOAP Note : (floor pts, if complex, use ICU PN)
S: patient reports: past problems, new problems, +/- anticipated problems
O: Vitals (Tmax, Pulse, BP, RR, pulse Ox)
    I/O: totals over past 24hrs or 8hrs, IVFs/ oral, urine, stool
    Wt: current and the trend
    PE: MS, CV, Resp, Abd, change from previous exam
    Labs: new results
    Meds: current
A/P: 1. Problem#1 discussion, assessment, and treatment plan.
     2. Problem#2 discussion, assessment, and treatment plan.

Discharge Note:
1) Date of admission/discharge
2) Diagnosis of admission/discharge
3) Attending and service to which pt. was admitted
4) Referring physician
5) Consultants: services and physicians
6) Procedures: date and indications (surgery, LPs, etc.)
7) Brief H&P with labs
8) Hospital Course
9) Disposition: discharged to where?
10) Discharge Meds
11) D/C Instructions and follow-up

Procedure Note (This is written after any procedure)
1) Procedure
2) Permit/Consent – benefits/risks/alternatives/signed/in chart
3) Indications
4) Physician(s)
5) Description of procedure
6) Complications
7) EBL
8) Disposition - pt. tolerated procedure well and ordered to remain supine 4-6 hrs.

48

Pre-Op Note
1) Pre-op diagnosis
2) Procedure planned
3) Indications for procedure
4) Lab results
5) CXR
6) EKG
7) Blood - type and crossed for 2 U PRBC
8) Orders – NPO, abx, skin/colon prep
9) Permit - Procedure described to patient, along with risks and benefits explained, consent signed, witnessed, and in chart.

Operative Note (PPP SAFE DCCS)
1) Pre-op Dx
2) Post-op Dx
3) Procedure
4) Surgeons
5) Anesthesia
6) Findings
7) EBL / Fluids/ urine output
8) Drains
9) Complications
10) Disposition/Condition
11) Specimens

ICU Rounds Presentation Sequence (presentation to Attendings)
1. PT summary
2. Overnight events
3. Vitals
4. Vent settings
5. ABG
6. I/O
7. MS
8. PE
9. Labs
10. Cx
11. Studies
12. A/P

Evening Rounds checklist (advance patients ASAP)
Vitals, I/O [UO], Eat?, BM?, OOB?
IVF dc? O2 dc? Abx dc? ADAT? Foley/tubes dc? Wound? (sutures/staples out?)
  # IVs (overnight access issues)
Orders: Am labs?
Look at: Notes / Plan of Care / Consults / Med list (IV→PO? stop? Drug levels?) /
  Studies/Cultures
DC planning: Social: Home/hosp/rehab/NH/LTAC, medical

ICU PN Efficient Smart Card
Overnight: main events which happened over night [hypotensive episodes, dysrhythmias]
  Subjective: Sleep? N/V/F/C/CP/SOB/Lightheaded? Pain? Bleeding? Flatus? BM?
Vitals: Tmax   T   BP   P   RR O_2sat%   End tital CO_2[inc?dec? ranges]
Neuro: [A&Ox3], sedation meds, *respond to voice? pain?* PEARRL, CNs, strength, DTRs, sensation, cerebellum, rectal
tone
Pulm: RR, O_2sat% #L O_2/RA. ET tube/ tracheostomy. chest tube [leak/ waterseal], secretions? *B L BS, wheezing,*
crackles, rhonchi, inspiration< expiration   **Vent settings:** [AC/SIMV/CPAP]/ rate/ TV/ PEEP/PS/ FiO2%
$(V_E=TV*RR)$
                          ABG for the vent: time/ pH/ pCO2/ pO2/ HCO3/ O2%/base +/- (PaO_2/FiO_2)
CV: Pressors, BP[range], P[range], End tital CO_2[inc?dec? ranges], CVP, Troponin I, EKG, ECHO, *S1, S2, RRR,*
murmur, rubs, JVD, pulses, edema **Swan-Ganz**[CO,CI,SVR]
GI/FEN: Diet[NPO(D#)/sips/clears/low fiber/regular], Tube feeds [type, rate, D#, total/residual], TPN[D#], *Stoma?*
Wounds? NG/OG/G/J tube? BM? (last one) Flatus? +BS, soft, NT, ND, bruits, masses, rebound, guarding,
hepatosplenomegaly, BRBPR, melana **I/O:** I (IVF[type,rate], TPN[rate], Tube[rate], PO[total])/ O (urine, NGT(#,#,#),
ostomy, JP#1(#,#,#,color)), **I=O?**
GU/Renal: urine: rate [ml/kg/hr], *urine color*
Heme/Onc: *lymphadnopathy, ecchymosis, petechia, SCDs?*
ID: Tmax, T, *wounds ulcers (C D I, dehiscence, erythema, pus), mouth lesions, lines infected?* Lines in: type, day#;
Vanco/gentamycin[peak,trough]

Meds: **Glu:**(last 24 hrs)[time, level, amt of insulin given]
Labs: BMP/ Ca+Mg+PO4 / CBC / coags   **Cx:**[site,date,result]
Studies: [CXR, ABD decub & lateral, KUB, EKG, CT, MRI, ECHO][include your impression]

A/P age, gender, relevant PMH POD# s/p what operation and an overview of the main problems. [why is this patient still
in the ICU? Everything can't be 'stable']

Neuro: Assessment: what sedation? GCS/Riker. A&Ox3? Respond to voice? pain? pupillary response? "follows
commands","moves all four ext." epidural? Cervical collar? ventriculostomy. Plan:[stable, CT, Rx ICP, freq neuro
checks, steroids, C/T/L precautions]. (agitated +HTN=OH withdrawal) Neurosurgery?

Pulm: Assessment:: (pneumonia, ARDS, COPD, pulmonary edema, CHF w/fluid overload). intubated/extubated D#? V_E,
PaO_2/FiO_2, ready for extubation? CXR results. Plan: what is being done (abx day#, ↓TV/↑PEEP, weaning plans, spO2%
91-92%, IPPB, ISB, suctioning, ipratropium, albuterol,steroids, etc.). CXR in am? Pulmonary?

CV: Assessment: NSR, afib, dysrhythmias, HTN (hypo/normo), CHF, cardiomyopathy. Controlled or not. Plan: Fluids?
pressors? HTN meds? Anti-Dysrhythmia meds?, Cardiology?

GI/FEN: Assessment: (ileus, pSBO) Plan: await return of bowel function, Tube feed: type, rate, total in/GR (8°). TPN.
on what prophylaxis[stop when eating]? (i.e.,colace, tagament, pepcid, zantac, carafate, protonix, senekot) Assessment:
Electrolytes (hyper/hypo). Plan: replace prn, labs in am? Assessment: Malnourished (Albumin)? Calorie goal. At goal?
Weight (admission weight). advance tube feeds? I=O?

GU/Renal: Assessment: urine output rate (Volume control: stable, oligouria, polyuria), BUN/Cr (azotemia↑/↑,uremia).
Prerenal([oligouria,>15,UNa↓],↓CO, hypovol, sepsis)/renal(Interstitial nephritis[↑Cr, oligouria,
F,eosin,hemat&proteinuria], usu 15 days after PCN, NSAIDS,diuretics exposure), ATN(UNa↑,1st oligouria[40-
400QD],↑BUN, 2nd ↑K, ↑H, ↑H₂O;hypotension, shock, sepsis, hemorrhage, myoglobinuria, gentamicin), Nephrotic
syn(proteinuria, hypoalbuminemia, edema), Nephritic syn(oliguria, azotemia, HTN, hematuria(red cell casts), mild
proteinuria/edema)/post renal failure (auria). Cr clearance? Plan: ↑IVFs, check FeNa, UA, ? Meds adjusted for renal
failure? Nephrology?

Heme/Onc: Assessment: leucocytosis, anemia, thrombocytosis, anticoagulated, coagulopathic, HIT? Plan: prophylaxis
(heparin, lovonox, SCDs, IVC Filter, none, ASA, plavix, coumadin). FeSO4, erythropoietin, MVI, Folate 1mg, thiamine
100mcg qd. Hematology?

ID: Assessment: (line-/uro-)Sepsis. Bacteremia, UTI. infection nidus, culture of that source, better/worse (trends Tmax,
WBC). Plan: Rx? change lines? Check UA C&S results? Abx D#? Infectious Disease?

ENDO: Assessment: DM? Ret cortisol deficiency? Glucose controlled? TSH level. ACTH suppression test. Plan:
Insulin gtt? ISS? NPH? start back on home meds. Endocrine?

Social: Assessment: DNR/DNI/Full code. Plan: Comfort care. Family notified of events?

50

Intensive Care

The ICU is a learning goldmine! This is where the really sick patients reside. I highly recommend taking an ICU elective during your senior year. Perhaps later in M3 year you might feel up to following a patient or two in 'the unit' during surgery or medicine. Remember as a resident you will follow patients in the ICU at some point. By doing a month in the unit your senior year, you will validate your understanding of all systems in the body. Anything you don't fully understand will come out for you to see. Each patient has many different things going on all at the same time. Caring for 1 patient in the unit is like 10 patients on the floor, with greater learning potential from the unit patient. It's a challenging experience, well worth your time taking the elective from a learning stand point. And it will give you the confidence to care for patients during your internship year.

Tools of the ICU

Cardiac monitor: provide a constant tracing of the heart activity. This is not a substitute for a 12 lead EKG. For cardiac evaluation always get a 12 lead EKG.

Arterial line/"A-line": An IV catheter in an artery (usually radial) that provides a continuous BP reading along with a site for arterial blood gases to be drawn rather than sticking the patient each day.

IV's: Intravenous access for fluids, meds, etc.

Central lines: IV's lines that go into central veins (femoral, subclavian, jugular).

Swan Ganz: a yellow catheter placed into the subclavian or jugular vein into the heart and pulmonary artery used for monitoring a patient's hemodynamic status. See Scut Monkey's Handbook.

Ventilator: Don't touch! Residents are not allowed to touch it. Only respiratory therapy can touch the vent.. See the section on the vent below.

Foley: a catheter placed in the bladder to accurately quantify hourly urinary output.

Chest tube: a tube inserted into the chest drain air or fluids from the pleural space.

Nasogastric (NG) tube: for draining things from (GI bleeds or to decompress the GI track when obstructed) or putting things in (feeding intubated patients) the stomach.

Dobhoff Tube: NG tube that goes to the duodenum (NGT goes to the stomach). For feeding when you want to bypass the stomach.

Oxygen: given by non-rebreather face mask or a nasal cannula.

TPN line: total parenteral nutrition. Used to feed the patient through a central line to maintain their nutritional requirements. This is often associated with Candida blood infections, so be careful.

Other drains: Read the OP-Note to find out where it connects to and its purpose.

Drips: IV medications to maintain blood pressure (dopamine), urine output (furosemide) or sedation (Versed) or pain/sedation (Morphine).

Data Collection

Unit patients have tons of data which has to collected, sorted and assimilated. There are several areas to look each morning. The nursing chart records hourly orders, vital signs, vent. settings, ABGs, daily weights, I's and O's (inputs and outputs from all sources), Swan-Ganz readings, rhythm, and medications. The main chart is for the H&P, all progress notes (from consulting physicians also), studies done and all other data not in the nursing chart. The computer provides up to date results on all labs.

ICU H&P General Format

CC: system failure responsible for admission to the ICU
HPI: (Include previous functional status prior to admission)
Brief Hospital course: Why did the pt come to the ICU or operation performed?
PMH:
SH: Smoke, Alcohol, Drugs
Allergies: to contrast? To pain meds?
Medications (outpatient):
Medications (at transfer):
Studies:

PE
Vitals: Tmax   T   BP   P   RR   Wt
Vent settings: vent setting/rate/TV/PEEP/ FiO2
ABG for the vent: pH/pCO2/pO2/HCO3/O2%
I/O:
Mental Status: on what for sedation? GCS description
HEENT:
Pulm:
CV:
Abd:
Rectal:
Ext:
Neuro:
Skin:

Labs:
CBC, BMP+ Mg/PO4/Ca, PT/PTT/INR
Cultures

Studies:
CXR
EKG

A/P overview of all main problems
Problem list by systems:
Neuro: on what sedation?
Pulm: intubated/extubated?
CV: on what pressors?
GI/FEN: on what prophylaxis?
GU/Renal:
Heme/Onc: on what prophylaxis?
ID:
Social: Family notified?

Morning Rounds Presentation/ Sequence for Progress Note

Sequence: 1. PT summary 2. Overnight events 3. Vitals 4. Vent settings 5. ABG 6. I/O
7. MS 8. PE 9. Labs 10. Cx 11. Studies 12. A/P

Details:

PT Summary: give the age, gender, relevant PMH and an overview of the main ICU problems the patient has (1-2 sentence, quick, short). The purpose of this is to remind everyone of the pt's story.

Overnight: main events which happened over night

Vitals: give ranges of vitals if they vary a lot over night (i.e., O_2sat 82-99%)

Vent: current settings

ABG: ABG for the current vent settings

I/O: total in and out for the last 24hrs, urine output per hour (per hr avg over last 8 hours), IV fluid type and rate per hr, rate of tube feeds and type: total amount and the gastric residual, GR, for the previous 8 hrs (With the GR the nurse sucks back on the NGT to see what is leftover in the stomach), weight, BM?.

PE

MS: amount of sedation meds and does the patient respond to voice or pain? (or Alert & Ox3)

HEENT: PEARRL, bruits, JVD, ear discharge, nose discharge, mouth lesions/infection

Pulm: B/L BS, wheezing, crackles, rhonchi, inspiration=expiration

CV: S1S2, S3, S4, RRR, murmur, rubs

Abd: soft, NT, ND, bruits, masses, rebound, guarding, hepatosplenomegaly, tympanic

Rectal: gross blood, masses, tone, guaiac,

Ext: pulses, edema

Neuro: CNs, strength, DTRs, sensation, cerebellum

Skin: ecchymosis, petechia, are lines going into patient not infected?

Labs: BMP+Mg/PO4/Ca, CBC with neutrophils/bands%, PT/PTT/INR (list also what it was previously or what the patient's baseline was)

Cx: look at old culture results everyday

Studies: CT, MRI, ECHO, CXR

A/P over all summary: age, gender, relevant PMH and an overview of the main ICU problems.

Problem list by systems:

Neuro: on what sedation? A&Ox3 or how does the pt respond to voice or pain?

Pulm: intubated/extubated Day#? CXR results. Lung problems (pneumonia, ARDS, COPD, etc) and what is being done (abx day#, ↓TV/↑PEEP, spO2% 91-92% with nebs, etc.). Vent setting, ABG and how you would like to change the settings.

CV: on what pressors? On HTN meds? Controlled or not.

GI/FEN: Tube feed: type, rate, total in/GR (8°). BM today? Last one? on what prophylaxis? (i.e.,colace, protonix, etc.) Glucose control over last 24°.

GU/Renal: Urine output rate. BUN/Cr.

Heme/Onc: WBC stable? HGB stable? PLT Stable? on what prophylaxis? (i.e., heparin, SCDs, etc.)

ID: list infection nidus, culture of that source, antibiotic day# for that source, better/worse (Tmax, WBC, etc.). What is being done for Tx?

Social: DNR/DNI status. Family notified of events?

ICU PN Efficient Smart Card

Overnight: main events which happened over night [hypotensive episodes, dysrhythmias]

Subjective: Sleep? N/V/F/C/CP/SOB/Lightheaded? Pain? Bleeding? Flatus? BM?

Vitals: Tmax T   BP   P   RR O_2sat%   End tital CO_2[inc?dec? ranges]

Neuro: [*A&Ox3*], sedation meds, *respond to voice? pain? PEARRL, CNs, strength, DTRs, sensation, cerebellum, rectal tone*

Pulm: RR, O_2sat% #L O_2/RA. ET tube/ tracheostomy. chest tube [leak/ waterseal], secretions? *B L BS, wheezing, crackles, rhonchi, inspiration< expiration* **Vent settings:** [AC/SIMV/CPAP]/ rate/ TV/ PEEP/PS/ FiO2% (V_E=TV*RR)

ABG for the vent: time/ pH/ pCO2/ pO2/ HCO3/ O2%/base +/- (PaO_2/FiO_2)

CV: Pressors, BP[range], P[range], End tital CO_2[inc?dec? ranges], CVP, Troponin I, EKG, ECHO, *S1, S2, RRR, murmur, rubs, JVD, pulses, edema* **Swan-Ganz**[CO,CI,SVR]

GI/FEN: Diet[NPO(D#)/sips/clears/low fiber/regular], Tube feeds [type, rate, D#, total/residual], TPN[D#], *Stoma? Wounds? NG/OG/G/J tube? BM? (last one) Flatus? +BS, soft, NT, ND, bruits, masses, rebound, guarding, hepatosplenomegaly, BRBPR, melana* **I/O:** I (IVF[type,rate], TPN[rate], Tube[rate], PO[total])/ **O** (urine, NGT(#,#,#), ostomy, JP#1(#,#,#,color)), **I=O?**

GU/Renal: urine: rate [ml/kg/hr], *urine color*

Heme/Onc: *lymphadnopathy, ecchymosis, petechia, SCDs?*

ID: Tmax, T, *wounds/ulcers (C/D I,dehiscence, erythema, pus), mouth lesions, lines infected?* Lines in: type, day#; Vanco/gentamycin[peak,trough]

Meds: **Glu:**(last 24 hrs)[time, level, amt of insulin given]
Labs: BMP/ Ca+Mg+PO4 / CBC / coags   **Cx:**[site,date,result]
Studies: [CXR, ABD decub & lateral, KUB, EKG, CT, MRI, ECHO][include your impression]

A/P age, gender, relevant PMH POD# s/p what operation and an overview of the main problems. [why is this patient still in the ICU? Everything can't be 'stable']

Neuro: Assessment: what sedation? GCS/Riker. A&Ox3? Respond to voice? pain? pupillary response? "follows commands","moves all four ext." epidural? Cervical collar? ventriculostomy. Plan:[stable, CT, Rx ICP, freq neuro checks, steroids, C/T/L precautions]. (agitated +HTN=OH withdrawal) Neurosurgery?

Pulm: Assessment:: (pneumonia, ARDS, COPD, pulmonary edema, CHF w/fluid overload). intubated/extubated D#? V_E, PaO_2/FiO_2, ready for extubation? CXR results. Plan: what is being done (abx day#, ↓TV/↑PEEP, weaning plans, spO2% 91-92%, IPPB, ISB, suctioning, ipratropium, albuterol,steroids, etc.). CXR in am? Pulmonary?

CV: Assessment: NSR, afib, dysrhythmias, HTN (hypo/normo), CHF, cardiomyopathy. Controlled or not. Plan: Fluids? pressors? HTN meds? Anti-Dysrhythmia meds?, Cardiology?

GI/FEN: Assessment: (ileus, pSBO) Plan: await return of bowel function, Tube feed: type, rate, total in/GR (8°). TPN. on what prophylaxis[stop when eating]? (i.e.,colace, tagament, pepcid, zantac, carafate, protonix, senekot) Assessment: Electrolytes (hyper/hypo). Plan: replace prn, labs in am? Assessment: Malnourished (Albumin)? Calorie goal. At goal? Weight (admission weight). advance tube feeds? I=O?

GU/Renal: Assessment: urine output rate (Volume control: stable, oligouria, polyuria), BUN/Cr (azotemia↑/↑,uremia). Prerenal([oligouria,>15,UNa↓],↓CO, reynold, sepsis)/renal(Interstitial nephritis[↑Cr, oligouria, F,eosin,hemat&proteinuria], usu 15 days after PCN, NSAIDS,diuretics exposure), ATN(UNa↑,1st oligouria[40-400QD],↑BUN, 2nd ↑K, ↑H, ↑H2O;hypotension, shock, sepsis, hemorrhage, myoglobinuria, gentamicin), Nephrotic syn(proteinuria, hypoalbuminemia, edema), Nephritic syn(oliguria, azotemia, HTN, hematuria(red cell casts), mild proteinuria/edema)/post renal failure (auria). Cr clearance? Plan: ↑IVFs, check FeNa, UA, ? Meds adjusted for renal failure? Nephrology?

Heme/Onc: Assessment: leucocytosis, anemia, thrombocytosis, anticoagulated, coagulopathic, HIT? Plan: prophylaxis (heparin, lovonox, SCDs, IVC Filter, none, ASA, plavix, coumadin). FeSO4, erythropoietin, MVI, Folate 1mg, thiamine 100mcg qd. Hematology?

ID: Assessment: (line-/uro-)Sepsis. Bacteremia. UTI. infection nidus. culture of that source, better/worse (trends Tmax, WBC). Plan: Rx? change lines? Check UA C&S results? Abx D#? Infectious Disease?

ENDO: Assessment: DM? Relative cortisoid deficiency? Glucose controlled? TSH level. ACTH suppression test. Plan: Insulin gtt? ISS? NPH? start back on home meds. Endocrine?

Social: Assessment: DNR/DNI/Full code. Plan: Comfort care. Family notified of events?

Ventilator Primer

Rule #1 Medical students and residents are not allowed to touch the ventilator, you might kill the patient! (only fellows and the respiratory therapist may touch the ventilator.)

Indications for putting a patient on a ventilator
1. Hypoxemic: (usu try 100% non-rebreather first, then CPAP, then on a ventilator)
2. Airway protection: (head trauma)
3. Inadequate ventilation (respiratory acidosis):
   A. Normal lungs (diaphragm paralysis, neuromuscular dz [Guillain-Barre syn, Polio, botulism], CNS depression (too much sedation), bleeds, kyphoscoliosis)
   B. Abnormal lungs (Asthma, COPD, ARDS)
4. Shock: (to decrease the work of breathing/save cardiac output)
5. Other: a. ↓ Intracranial Pressure via hyperventilation
   b. Flail chest

Ventilator Terms
Ventilators: positive pressure inflation of lungs (physiologic is negative pressure)

Modes:
Volume control
AC Assist Control: Pt is sedated. Pt triggered, vent delivers a fixed TV (a minimum RR & TV are set, if the pt doesn't trigger an inspiration). Most commonly used mode.
CMV Control Mode Ventilation: Pt must be sedated and paralyzed. Vent provides RR & TV (pt not allowed to participate).
IMV Intermittent Mandatory Ventilation: Pt is allowed to breath unassisted in between machine breaths.
SIMV Synchronized Intermittent Mandatory Ventilation: Pt gets the set RR & TV + whatever the pt initiates & the volume the pt can pull.

Pressure control
PSV Pressure Support Ventilation: Pt determines PIFR, insp/exp & RR. More comfort. Pressures of 5, 10, 15, 20: often used as a weaning mode. No back up RR if the pt stops breathing. (same as CPAP except pt is intubated and on the vent)
PCV Pressure Control Ventilation: Vent controls PIFR, RR.

APRV Airway Pressure Release Ventilation: relatively new mode of ventilation. Produces TV ventilation using a release of airway pressure from an elevated baseline to produce a simulated expiration.

Advantages:
- Elevated baseline facilitates oxygenation
- Timed releases aid in carbon dioxide removal
- Lower airway pressures
- Lower minute ventilation
- Minimal adverse effects on cardiac output
- May spontaneously breathe

APRV settings
  P High: Upper airway pressure
  P Low: Lower airway pressure
  T High: time which P High is maintained
  T low: time which P low is maintained

Patients usu are not weaned off the vent from this mode.

Note: for more info see the above reference – a nice review of theory and practice.

FiO$_2$: Percent of oxygen delivered by vent. Room air is 21%. Usually initially 90-100%.
Move in increments ASAP to FiO$_2$<50% and PaO$_2$ 60-80mmHg to avoid O$_2$ toxicity.

TV Tital Volume: Amount of gas delivered in each respiratory cycle.
Normal lungs: 10-12 ml/kg (of ideal body weight, not real body weight).
Diseased lungs (COPD/ARDS): 4-6 ml/kg for best results.

Other ideas about PEEP & TV adjustment: real time Pressure Volume curve on vent. Look at
lower and upper inflection points. Lower inflection point +2 should be where PEEP is set. TV
should not exceed the upper inflection point (or you are causing barotrauma).

PIFR Peak Inspiratory Flow Rate: (how fast to give the inspiration)
Usually 50-60 L/min (4 times the resting minute volume, MV)
If obstructed (COPD) pushing in faster 90-100L/min allows more time to exhale.
If restricted (ARDS) 30-50L/min (limit peak inspiration pressure).

Trigger: Usually 0.5-1.0 cm H$_2$0
Goal: to trigger inspiration with the least amount of pt effort without causing auto-cycling.

Waveform:

      Square: (for COPD)   Descending: (for ARDS)

PEEP:
Indications: Pt with hypoxemia despite FiO$_2$ of 50% or more. ↓work in COPD pts.
Contraindications (relative): unilateral lung dz, PTX, bronchopleural fistula, hypovolemia,
↑ ICP, cardiac shunt, some COPD/Asthma pts.
Normal: +5 is physiologic (the glottis produces this).
Theory: +5 prevents alveolar collapse, opens previous closed alveoli.
Problems using PEEP: ↓Cardiac output (also ↓renal & portal blood flow), barotrauma, ↑ICP
(high levels). Overcome CO problem via (fluids & pressors).
Goals: Keep PEEP at a minimum such that PaO$_2$>60 with FiO$_2$ <50%.
Initially: give +5 (including COPD). Usually go up by +2.5. +15 - +20 is the area where
PTX tends to happen.
Using PEEP: If PEEP >10 and pt has cardiac dz, you should monitor pulmonary artery
wedge pressures, PAW. (PEEP>10 PAW overestimates LV filling pressures, disconnect vent
for 3 sec and get accurate PAW – but note below what happens upon suddenly stopping
PEEP).

Adjusting PEEP:

↑ **PEEP:** go up +2.5 at a time (remember this can cause barotrauma; PTX). After ↑ PEEP, full results will be seen in about 4 hours. Goal: ↑ until PaO_2>60 with FiO_2 <50%.

↓ **PEEP:** go down +2.5 at a time. Watch for Δ in BP, HR, and RR (you will see results with in a minute, if not seconds). Draw ABG after 20 min. If PaO_2>60 on the new PEEP, continue to drop PEEP (not faster that +5 Q6°). Pts taking the last step to +5 is an often the hardest step (post extubation might require CPAP mask). If pt starts to desaturate O_2 then, switch settings to FiO_2 100% & PEEP back to the previous setting, get ABG and start again to work towards decreasing FiO_2 back down as far as possible, allow pt to rest a day or so, then reattempt dropping PEEP again).

Other ideas about PEEP & TV adjustment: real time Pressure Volume curve on vent. Look at lower and upper inflection points. Lower inflection point +2 should be where PEEP is set. TV should not exceed the upper inflection point (or you are causing barotrauma).

RR, Rate: usually at least 12 bpm. <12 bpm used for COPD pts to ↑ exhalation time (if greater, autoPEEP may result). >20 bpm for ARDS pts with low TV, thus meeting minute volume requirements (also for ↓ ICP).

Type of face mask modes (related topic: not ventilator terms)
These are typically for cooperative, conscious, hypercapnic COPD pts.
CPAP: A constant pressure, all the time. Pt must initiate the breath.
BIPAP: A constant pressure & increased pressure during inspiration. Pt must initiate.

Theory: Normal people, to inspire: expand chest, ΔV … -2mmHg ΔP created … air flows in because atmosphere, atm P = 0. COPD pts rest at +10mmHg, so to inspire: expand chest, ΔV … to get to -2mmHg for air to flow in, extra movement of chest must occur to generate ΔP = -12 for air to flow in. CPAP makes the pt's atmosphere +10 (to meet the pt's baseline of +10). So now the pt can breathe like a normal person. To inspire: pt's baseline +10, pt expands chest, +8 is reached in the lungs. Since atm is +10, air flows in and the pt only uses energy to change the chest volume to produce ΔP = 2 (like a normal person). Draw backs of CPAP: GI hyperinflation, necrosis of ears & nose from mask, eating is difficult.

Getting started with the Ventilator (usually)
In General: Intubate, listen for breath sounds, stat pCXR, stat ABG, end tital CO_2 measure. Set initial vent settings. Look at pCXR, is ET tube 4-5cm above carina? Possibly reposition ET tube. Look at ABG, readjust the vent. Get another ABG 20 min, readjust vent (if O2 sat and pulse oximetry are correlating, and end tital CO2 monitor and CO2 on ABG correlate, then repeat ABGs are not necessary). Repeat over and over trying to reach a goal of PaO_2>60mmHg, FiO_2<50%. Minimize oxygen toxicity as fast as possible (that's why you repeat ABG Q 20-30 min).

1. Normal lungs
FiO_2: 90-100% (move soon to <50% to avoid O_2 toxicity; PaO_2 60-80mmHg)
Mode: AC
Trigger: flow/pressure
TV: 10-12 ml/kg
PIFR: 60 L/min
PEEP: +5 is physiologic
RR: 12-18 bpm

2. Asthma/COPD
FiO_2 90-100% (move soon to <50% to avoid O_2 toxicity; PaO_2 60-80mmHg)
Mode: AC
Trigger: flow/pressure
TV: 4-6 ml/kg
PIFR: 90-100L/min (push in fast so each cycle will have more time to exhale)
Waveform: Square
PEEP: +5 is physiologic
RR: <12

3. ARDS (alveolar flooding/atelectasis/normal lung with areas of dense consolidation)
FiO_2 90-100% (move soon to <50% to avoid O_2 toxicity; PaO_2 60-80mmHg)
Mode: AC
Trigger: flow/pressure
TV: keep low, 4-6 ml/kg (pCO_2 60 is OK "permissive hypercapnia)
PIFR: keep lower. 40L/min (high inspiration, lower expiration)
Waveform: Descending
PEEP: start +5, go up by 2.5 increments. ↑ alveoli opening and functioning, ↓ venous return, ↓ Cardiac output, ↓ oxygen delivery. 15-20 = possible PTX

After Setup
1. Obstructive: Asthma/COPD
Goal: Supportive.
Theory: COPD pts get tired by working hard for days before coming to the hospital. These pts have difficulty exhaling (they actually have to expend energy exhaling!) and retain volume/CO_2, so each breath cycle results in less alveolar ventilation, so they develop hypercapnia.
(Aside: when obstructive pts are not allowed to exhale fully, they retain a little volume with each breath. Intrathoracic pressure ↑…venous return of blood ↓…cardiac output ↓ … hypotension … shock! This can happen if an obstructive pt is ambu bagged too fast (or ventilated) and not allowed to fully exhale (called 'autoPEEP'). Tx: Stop bagging or disconnect the vent. and allow the pt to exhale! (within 1 min BP will return).
Permissive hypercapnia is OK as long as goal is to give bronchodilators and the pt is allowed to exhale and rest.
Strategy: Limiting plateau pressure <35, peak pressures up to 70 are usu well tolerated, prolonging lung expiration helps the lungs to empty (either low TV <10cc/kg, high peak flow >60L/min, or low RR <12-16bpm), square waveform.

2. ARDS/ B/L pneumonia
Goal: To open alveoli by keeping TV low and PEEP high.
Theory: a PEEP of +8 - +15 lungs will start to open alveoli; ARDS is shunt physiology.
How to get there: Increase PEEP 2.5 at a time (remember this can cause barotrauma; PTX)
How long to see a response: After increasing PEEP, results will be seen in about 4 hours.
Reducing PEEP by 2.5 and you will see results in seconds. If the pt starts to desaturate O_2 then switch settings to FiO_2 100% & PEEP back to the previous setting, get ABG and work to decrease FiO_2 back down as far as possible, before attempting to change PEEP again.
Strategy: Involves trying to keep plateau pressure <35 & prolong inspiration time (low TV, low peak flow rates <50 L/min, descending waveform, RR up to 30 bpm).

Evaluating patients on the Vent. (daily)
(MV) Minute Volume: MV=RR* TV (report minute volume daily in rounds)
<10 good: Pt doing well.
>15 bad: Pt not doing well. (sick pts will have a high MV)

(PAP) Peak Airway Pressure: PAP = resistance of airways +resistance of lung parenchyma
(PP) Plateau Pressure = resistance of lung parenchyma
PAP: <50 is ideal
              >60-70 not good; look at the PP

PP: normal lungs =30
              <35 (ddx: mucus plug, kink in the tube/pt biting the tube, bronchospasm)
              Suction: never insert while suction is on (it can cause tracheal bleeding)
              >35 lung injury, get stat CXR (ddx: PTX; especially suspect if a procedure was
previously done or if PEEP is $\geq$ +15) If PTX on CXR + hypotension => insert a 16 gauge
needle into 2nd intercostals space as it is a tension PTX (or notify your resident/attending).
RR: < 30 should be less than this
              >30 something is not right

Compliance: $\Delta V/\Delta P$ (measure of lung stiffness)
To calculate compliance: you need plateau pressure (obtained by adding an inspiratory pause
to the respiratory cycle on the vent), peak airway pressure and TV.

SC, Static Compliance: elastic properties of lung ($\downarrow$by:interstitial fibrosis/edema, alveolar
flooding ddx: PTX, atelectasis, worsening pneumonia, pulmonary edema)
SC=TV/(PP-PEEP) [normal: 60-100 ml/cmH2O]

DC, Dynamic Compliance: elastic & resistive properties($\downarrow$ by ddx: bronchospasm, ET tube
kinking, excessive secretions)
DC=TV/(PAP-PEEP) [normal: 50-80 ml/cmH20]

Exhale TV: in = out unless there is a leak. Deflate the cuff and see that in $\neq$ out.

Weaning (Wean & extubate ASAP)
(cumulated incidence of nosocomial pneumonia D3: 8%, D7: 21%, D14: 32%, >D14: 45%).

Conditions required before trying to wean
1. Recovery from the cause of respiratory failure
2. Cessation of sedation
3. Off pressors (such as norepinephine)
4. Alert, cooperative pt who can cough for you.
5. Corrected metabolic disorders
6. Adequate gas exchange:
        a. PaO_2/FiO_2>200
        b. PaO_2>60mmHg, FiO_2<50%, PEEP$\leq$+5cm H_2O
        c. PaO_2/PAO_2>0.35
7. Best predictor of successful weaning: Pt on the T-piece, measure RSBI=RR/TV (liters):
RSBI <80 good candidate to extubate
RSBI 80-100 proceed but be careful
RSBI >105 pt not ready, wait longer
(even with all positive predictors, 20% of extubated pts will fail and have to be reintubated)

Method

1. Spontaneous Breathing Trial. Place pt on a T-piece.
2. Observe pt for 30 min (stand at bedside). Look for distress:
   a. Tachycardia/Bradycardia
   b. Hypertension/Hypotension
   c. Arrhythmias/PVCs
   d. Cyanosis/nasal alae flaring/sweating/pursed lips/struggled breaths
3. If distress, put pt back on vent and wait 24 hrs (let the pt rest) and reevaluate reasons why failed. Try again after 24hrs (QD trial of spontaneous breathing, gradually lengthing the trial).
4. If successful, get everything ready at bedside before extubation.
   a. Intubation kit (20% have to be reintubated)
   b. CPAP/100% O_2 nonrebreather with oxygen ready
   c. Suction
   d. Something for pt to spit mucus into.
   e. Respiratory therapy/the fellow/attending (in the event of reintubation)
5. Consult a text for more details on the hard pts to wean.

Examples:

1. 32♀ 5'4" 130lbs (60kg) with heroin induced Asthma attack. Intubated twice in the past. So she is intubated on the vent.: AC/20/300/+5/100% square waveform. 1st ABG 7.17/120/225/98%. So change the vent settings: AC/20/400/+5/80% with a ABG of 7.24/90/180/98%. So now you change vent. to AC/26/400/+5/60%. While your waiting 20 min to get the next ABG the nurse calls you saying the pt's BP is dropping! What did you do? autoPEEP is the answer. What should you do to fix the problem? Pull the vent tubing off the ET tube and allow the pt to exhale (to save the patient), the BP should go up. Now change the vent to ↑ PIFR to allow more time to exhale in each cycle.

2. Pt with bad B/L pneumonia (ARDS picture)
Pt is currently on PEEP +5 and FiO2 100% with 7.32/45/51. How should you change the vent? ↑ PEEP, this will help to open alveoli. High TV is detrimental to ARDS lungs. 6 ml/kg should be goal.

60

Weaning from vent

PaO$_2$/FiO$_2$

1. PaO$_2$/FiO$_2$>200
2. PaO$_2$>60mmHg, FiO$_2$<50%, PEEP≤+5cm H$_2$O

PaO$_{2[mmHg]}$ (if PaO2/FiO2<200 = ARDS)

FiO$_2$	50	60	70	80	90	100	110	120	130	140	150	160	170	180
0.2	250	300	350	400	450	500	550	600	650	700	750	800	850	900
0.3	167	200	233	267	300	333	367	400	433	467	500	533	567	600
0.4	125	150	175	200	225	250	275	300	325	350	375	400	425	450
0.5	100	120	140	160	180	200	220	240	260	280	300	320	340	360
0.6	83	100	117	133	150	167	183	200	217	233	250	267	283	300
0.7	71	86	100	114	129	143	157	171	186	200	214	229	243	257
0.8	63	75	88	100	113	125	138	150	163	175	188	200	213	225
0.9	56	67	78	89	100	111	122	133	144	156	167	178	189	200
1	50	60	70	80	90	100	110	120	130	140	150	160	170	180

Minute Ventilation [L/min]

MV=RR* TV

1. <10 good: Pt doing well
2. >15 bad: Pt not doing well (sick pts will have a high MV)

Normal lungs TV = 10-12 ml/kg (of ideal body weight)

ideal weight *10 RR

Height	lbs	kg	TV[ml]	8	9	10	11	12	13	14	15	16	17	18	19	20	21	22	23	24	25	26	27	28	29	30
5' 0"	120	54	544	4	5	5	6	7	7	8	8	9	9	10	10	11	11	12	13	13	14	14	15	15	16	16
5' 2"	130	59	590	5	5	6	6	7	8	8	9	9	10	11	11	12	12	13	14	14	15	15	16	17	17	18
5' 4"	140	63	635	5	6	6	7	8	8	9	10	10	11	11	12	13	13	14	15	15	16	17	17	18	18	19
5' 6"	150	68	680	5	6	7	7	8	9	10	10	11	11	12	12	13	14	14	15	16	16	17	18	18	19	20
5' 8"	160	73	726	6	7	7	8	9	9	10	11	11	12	12	13	14	15	15	16	17	17	18	19	20	20	21
5' 10"	170	77	771	6	7	8	8	9	10	11	12	12	13	14	15	15	16	17	18	19	19	20	21	22	22	23
6' 0"	180	82	816	7	7	8	9	10	11	11	12	13	14	15	16	16	17	18	19	20	20	21	22	23	24	24
6' 2"	190	86	862	7	8	8	9	10	11	12	13	14	15	16	16	17	18	19	20	20	21	22	22	23	24	25
6' 4"	200	91	907	7	8	9	10	11	12	13	14	15	15	16	17	18	19	20	21	22	23	24	24	25	26	27

COPD/ARDS lungs TV = 4-6 ml/kg (of ideal body weight)

ideal weight *6 RR

Height	lbs	kg	TV[ml]	12	13	14	15	16	17	18	19	20	21	22	23	24	25	26	27	28	29	30	31	32	33	34
5' 0"	120	54	327	4	4	5	5	5	6	6	6	7	7	7	8	8	8	9	9	9	10	10	10	11	11	
5' 2"	130	59	354	4	4	5	5	5	6	6	7	7	7	8	8	9	9	10	10	10	11	11	11	12	12	
5' 4"	140	63	381	5	5	5	6	6	6	7	7	8	8	9	9	10	10	10	11	11	11	12	12	13	13	
5' 6"	150	68	408	5	5	6	6	7	7	7	8	8	9	9	10	10	11	11	11	12	12	13	13	13	14	
5' 8"	160	73	435	5	6	6	7	7	7	8	8	9	9	10	10	11	11	12	12	13	13	14	14	14	15	
5' 10"	170	77	463	6	6	6	7	7	8	8	9	9	10	11	11	12	12	13	13	14	14	15	15	15		
6' 0"	180	82	490	6	6	7	7	8	8	9	9	10	10	11	11	12	12	13	13	14	14	15	15	16	16	17
6' 2"	190	86	517	6	7	7	8	8	9	9	10	10	11	11	12	12	13	13	14	14	15	16	16	17	17	18
6' 4"	200	91	544	7	7	8	8	9	9	10	10	11	11	12	13	13	14	14	15	15	16	17	17	18	18	19

PaO2 needed for an A-a gradient to be 10
(if PaO2 is less, then A-a gradient>10)

PaCO2

FiO2	10	15	20	25	30	35	40	45	50	55	60
0.21	130	125	120	115	110	105	100	95	90	85	80
0.3	194	189	184	179	174	169	164	159	154	149	144
0.4	265	260	255	250	245	240	235	230	225	220	215
0.5	337	332	327	322	317	312	307	302	297	292	287
0.6	408	403	398	393	388	383	378	373	368	363	358
0.7	479	474	469	464	459	454	449	444	439	434	429
0.8	550	545	540	535	530	525	520	515	510	505	500
0.9	622	617	612	607	602	597	592	587	582	577	572
1	693	688	683	678	673	668	663	658	653	648	643

	NC	FiO2	Venturi (for COPD)
	1 L/min	24%	24%
	2 L/min	28%	28%
	3 L/min	32%	
	4 L/min	36%	36%
	5 L/min	40%	40%
	6 L/min	44%	
	Face mask	60%	
	FM+reservoir: 6 L/min	60%	
	7 L/min	70%	
	8 L/min	80%	
	9 L/min	90%	
	10 L/min	95%	
	15 L/min	100%	

References:
1. Most of the following information was taught to me from attending physicians while on my MICU rotation at Cook County Hospital. I also obtained additional information from the Dept of Medicine MICU Curriculum Text at Cook County Hospital, Chicago, IL.
2. APRV: Frawley PM, Habashi, NM, Airway Pressure Release Ventilation: Theory and Practice, AACN Clinical Issues, Vol 12, Number 2, pp234-246.

Notes

EKG Primer

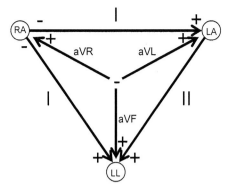

Steps in analyzing a EKG
(a systematic approach)

1. Scale & leads placed correctly?

2. Rate (Ventricular & Atrial)
3. P wave morphology & amplitude
4. Origin of rhythm

5. PR, QRS, QT intervals

6. QRS axis & voltage
7. Q waves?
8. R wave progression
9. ST segment
10. T wave
11. U wave
12. Baseline
13. Pacemaker

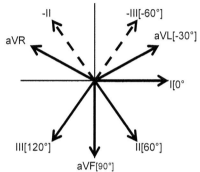

14. Arrythmias present?
15. Hypertrophy?
16. Ischemia, Injury, Infarction present?

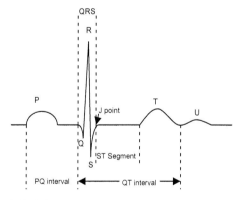

Groups of leads:
Inferior: II, III, aVF
Septal: V_{1-2}
Anterior: V_{2-4}
Lateral: V_{4-6}, I, aVL
R vent.:V_4 R wave
Posterior infarct if: voltage drops off
from V_{4-6} & V_1 has a large wide R

1 small box= 0.04 sec (40msec) and 1mm in height
1 large box=0.2sec (200msec) and 5mm in height

63

Scale & Leads placed correctly?

•Scale: On the left of the EKG the base line should make an upright rectangle 10 box high, this is normal. If 5 box high, then you will have to multiply all heights by 2.

•Lead Placement: P should be + in II; aVR should have a + R; P, QRS, T are all + in I, otherwise consider lead misplaced. ("white to right; smoke over fire")

Rate (ventricular) [normal 60-100]
• [Count large boxes from R to R: 300, 150, 100, 75, 60, And 50]
<60 Bradycardia
>100 Tachycardia
150-250 Paroxysmal Tachycardia
250-350 Flutter
350-450 Fibrillation

•Kids (upper normal limit): 0-1yr HR 180; 1-3yr 150; 4-10yr 130; 10yr+ 110;

P wave morphology & amplitude [look at II 1st;height<2.5bx; width<3bx]
•Morphology: Is it + or -? Is it biphasic(+ & -)? Is it present (yes/no)?
P should be + along II; if −, either leads misplaced or SA node is not the pacer (perhaps AV or atria ectopic foci are pacing)
•If biphasic see Hypertrophy section (RAH & LAH)
•If P is − in II consider leads misplaced (esp. if aVR has + R)

Origin of rhythm[atria, AV, ventricular]
Atria:
•P present? P before every QRS? =>P must be + in II for normal sinus rhythm [usu HR 60-80]
•Do all the Ps look the same? If not =>wandering atrial pacemaker (<100) or Multifocal Atrial Tachycardia (>100)
•Sawtooth pattern of Ps, followed by a QRS=>atrial flutter (usu with rapid vent. response)
AV node:
•No distinct Ps, Normal looking QRS ? => possibly AV node pacing [usu HR 40-60] or atrial fibrillation
Ventricle:
•PVC looking, QRS with wide inverted T wave without P waves?=>ventricular foci pacing [usu HR 20-40] (pacemakers look similar, electrode at the ventricular apex)

Is the rhythm regular? (if no, see Arrythmias present? Section)

PR, QRS, QT intervals

PR [use II: 3-5 box] (short/normal/long; constant/lengthening/variable)
•If PR >5box =>1° AV block

QRS [use longest lead;>2.5 box = wide](normal/wide)
•If wide, why? Look at leads:

	V1	I +V6
RBBB	'M-like' QRS	wide S
LBBB	wide S	wide R
IVCD	neither of the above, just wide QRS	
WPW	wide QRS, delta wave (PR curves into the QRS), short PR	

•Incomplete BBB = rSr' pattern (V_{1or2} for RBBB and V_{5or6} for LBBB)

•Note: Secondary ST-T wave changes for R/LBBB, ST-T is opposite of the final dir. of the terminal component of the QRS (i.e., if terminal cpt is a – S then the ST-T wave should be + or if the terminal cpt is a + R then the ST-T wave should be -).

Suspect infarction if: 1. New conduction delay in pt w/ chest pain
        2. LBBB: Q in I or V6
        3. RBBB: deep/wide Q in any leads
        4. Primary ST-T changes (opposite to the above Note)
•Acute RBBB => think PE

QT[the longest QT;usu <9.5 box; QT<1/2 R-R dist.; <500msec] (normal/prolonged)
•Note: Prolonged QT can cause sustained ventricular tachycardia which can cause hemodynamic collapse, therefore always check.
•Can cause prolonged QT: Hypocalcemia, Hypomagnesemia, hypokalemia
•Drugs that are generally accepted to prolong QT and/or Induce Torsades de Pointes Ventricular Arrhythmia (see www.qtdrug.org for updates):
Anti-arrhythmic:Amiodarone, Disopyramide, Dofetilide, Ibutilide, *Procainamide, Quinidine,* Sotalol
Antimicrobial: Chloroquine (malaria), Clarithromycin, *Erythromycin,* Halofantrine (malaria), *Pentamidine* (PCP), Sparfloxacin (Antibiotic)
Anti-psychotic:Chlorpromazine, *Haloperidol,* Mesoridazine, Pimozide, Thioridazine
GI:Cisapride (heartburn), Domperidone (Anti-nausea), Droperidol (Sedative;Anti-nausea)
Opiate agonist:Levomethadyl, Methadone
Other:Arsenic trioxide (Anti-cancer / Leukemia), Bepridil (Anti-anginal)

QRS axis & voltage

Axis:	leads:	I	aVF
Normal axis:		+	+
LAD:		+	-
RAD:		-	+
Indeterminate:		-	-

•Note: LAD is pathologic if lead II is (-) (axis < -30°) => think LAFB
•Normal axis for kids: 0-30d 180°; 30d-1yr 120°; 1yr-16yr 100°
•Hemiblock/Fascicle:
LAFB(L Anterior fascicle block): LAD + R wave of aVL before R wave of aVR or LAD + Q in 1 & S in 3
LPFB(L Posterior fascicle block): RAD + R wave of aVR before R wave of aVL or RAD + S1 Q3

Low QRS Voltage [total of 8 leads w/: precordial leads<10 bx or limb leads<5 bx]
•Note: Posterior infarct if: voltage drops off from V_{4-6} & V_1 has a large wide R
•ddx: Pericardia/pleural effusion, COPD, Cardiomyopathy, Cardiac infiltration (amyloidosis), Constrictive pericarditis, Tamponade, Hypothyroid (also see bradycardia), Obesity, Normal variant, Anasarca, Transplant (acute/chronic rejection), (L) PTX, MI, Myocarditis (acute/chronic), or Dilated cardiomyopathy (low limb & prominent precordial)

Q waves?
•Significant (pathologic) Q wave= 1box wide or 1/3 the height of the R wave
•Q wave = infarct in all leads except: (aVR; small in I, aVL, V_4-V_6; only 1 large Q in III, aVF, aVL, or V_1 is acceptable without an infarct being present)

Poor R wave progression [def. V_3 R<3 box]
•V_2-V_4 a transition should occur, if not consider the ddx below or MI.
•Tall R in V_1 + voltage drops off from V_{4-6} usu indicates Posterior infarct
•rSr' pattern in V_{1or2} = Incomplete LBBB
•ddx: leads misplaced, Septal or anterior MI, LVH, RVH, LBBB, LAHB, IVCD, COPD, Dextrocardia, WPW, Left PTX (R mediastinum shift), Ventricular aneurysm, or Pectus excavatum
•Tall R in V_1 (ddx: Posterior MI, RBBB, RVH, WPW, normal variant)

ST segment (any lead except aVR)
•ST seg elevation: Concave:Up "smiley"= good/ok (esp. if with a J point)
                    Concave down "frowny"= bad (usu acute injury)
•Elevation>1 box (2 or more leads) = injury
•Depression>1 box (2 or more leads) = ischemia
•Pericarditis: stage 1. everything is up (diffuse ST seg elev.) stage 2. everything is down (diffuse T inversion).

T wave [height<5bx,<10bx (precordial)]
•Inversion ok in: III, aVF, aVL, aVR + V_1
•Hyperkalemia: peaked T [renal failure or acidosis can cause ↑K]
•Ischemia: inverted isosceles triangle
•Strain: a downward sloping ST segment into an inverted T wave
•Non Specific ST-T abnormalities: flattening of T waves or biphasic
•Pericarditis: stage 1. everything is up (diffuse ST seg elev.) 2. everything is down (diffuse T inversion).

U wave: Present in: hypokalemia, LVH, or Bradycardia

Arrythmias present?
Sinus origin, Regular rhythm(P + in II)
•Normal Sinus Rhythm(NSR): HR 60-99
•Sinus Bradycardia:HR<60
•Sinus Tachycardia:HR ≥100

Sinus origin, Irregular rhythm (P + in II)
Sinus arrhythmia: either associated with respirations or not (common in kids).

Supraventricular (Narrow QRS)
•Atrial Fibrillation: no definite P waves; irregularly irregular rhythm with: Rapid vent. response: HR>120; Mod.: HR 70-110; Slow: HR<60
•Atrial Flutter:reg. atrial rate about 300; sawtooth pattern: HR 150(2:1) or 75(4:1)
• (PSVT)Paroxysmal SupraVentricular Tachycardia: usu an regular AV reentry tachycardia usu 150-240 (not obvious atrial activity or sometimes P – in II)
•Junctional(AV node) rhythms: regular, P – in II or absent
HR 40-60=>AV Node Escape rhythm (SA node is delayed)
HR 61-99=>Accelerated Junctional rhythm
HR 100+ =>Junctional Tachycardia

Premature beats: (happens before the time you would expect a beat to occur)
•P present, normal QRS=>premature atrial contraction (PAC)
•No P, normal looking QRS=> premature junctional contraction

•No P, not normal QRS w/ wide inverted T?=>premature ventricular contraction
•Escape beats: (happens after a pause)
-P present, normal QRS=>Atrial escape beat
-No P, normal looking QRS=> Junctional escape beat
-No P, not normal QRS w/ wide inverted T=>Ventricular escape beat

Ventricular (wide QRS) (arise from a focus in the ventricles)
Usu fairly regular rhythm with no P, not normal QRS w/ wide inverted T:
•HR 30-40 =>Idioventricular escape rhythm
•HR 50-120=>Accelerated Idioventricular rhythm
•HR 120+ =>Ventricular tachycardia
•HR totally disorganized, no peripheral pulse => Ventricular Fibrillation

Hypertrophy
LVH [any of the below]
•$R_{V5 \text{ or } 6}$ +$S_{V1 \text{ or } 2}$≥35 (in pts >35yr)
•R_I + S_{III} >25
•R_{AVL}>11
•R_{AVF}>14
•$R_{V5 \text{ or } V6}$>26

•Note suspect LVH if: RBBB: aVL≥12 or $R_{V5 \text{ or } 6}$≥25
                             LBBB: $S_{V1, 2 \text{ or } 3}$≥30
•Note: LVH more likely to be present with 'Strain'

RVH(don't try to diagnose if LBBB,RBBB, or IVCD)
•RAD≥110° (or indeterminate axis)
•R_{V1}≥7
•S_{V1}<2
•Suggestive of RVH: RAH, *RAD, incomplete RBBB, low voltage, persistent precordial S waves*, R ventricular strain, Tall R in V_1
•Note: *Findings suggestive of pulmonary disease in italics.*

RAH
•P≥2.5 box tall + peaked in II, III, aVF
•Biphasic; 1st part peeked/pointed (not curved) & 1 box can fit in the second component

LAH
•P≥3box wide + notched (M shaped) in I, II, aVL or
•Biphasic; 1st part curved (not peeked/pointed) & 1 full box can fit in the second component

General

- 'Strain': asymmetrical ST seg depression & T wave inversion (a downward sloping ST segment into an inverted T wave); or flat ST with flattening of T waves
- Timing of Infarction:
  - Acute(hrs-day): *ST seg. elevated & concave down*; Q absent/minimal; T inversion absent/minimal; or *ST depression*
  - Recent(day-week):*Q present*; ST seg absent/min; *T inversion present*; ST depression absent/minimal
  - Old(>week): *Q present*; ST seg absent/min; T inversion absent/min; ST depression absent
- COPD: If low voltage in lead I and R = S (axis is 90°) then pt most likely.
- PE: classic: wide S_1/ large Q_3/ $\perp_3$ + ST$\downarrow_2$, sinus tachycardia, V_1-$V_4{}^\perp$ with RBBB + ST$\downarrow_2$,
  - R axis deviation

References:
Cardiology elective, teachings from attending physicians at the Chicago Medical School
ECG Interpretation Pocket Reference, Ken Grauer, M.D., FAAFP
Rapid Interpretation of EKG's, Dale Dubin, M.D.

Acid-Base
(Arterial blood gas and venous electrolytes)

(Chem-7)Venous Electrolytes Anion Gap = Na – (HCO3 + Cl) [8-16]

Na	Cl	BUN	
135-145 mEq/L	98-106 mEq/L	7-18 mg/dL	Glucose
			70-115 mg/dL
K	HCO$_3$	Cr	
3.5-5.1 mEq/L	22-29 mEq/L	0.6-1.2 mg/dL	

Note: venous electrolytes are valuable, in that, they are usually readily available and can provide much information about the patient's acid base status fast, if you understand the patterns.

1. HCO$_3$ (bicarbonate): Used to evaluate metabolic acid-base & respiratory acid-base (via chronic renal compensation) disorders:
    a. HCO$_3$ low:
        i.   Metabolic acidosis or
        ii. Respiratory alkalosis with renal compensation.

    b. HCO$_3$ high:
        i.   Metabolic alkalosis or
        ii. Respiratory acidosis with renal compensation.

2. Anion Gap: Used to evaluate metabolic acidosis conditions
    a. Anion Gap = Na – (HCO$_3$ + Cl) [8-16]
    b. Anion Gap metabolic acidosis (normochloremic)
        i.   Most common disorders:
            1. Ketoacidosis
            2. Lactic acidosis
            3. Renal failure
        ii. Typical anion gaps
            1. Salicylates: nml→ 20
            2. Renal failure: nml→ 25
            3. DKA: nml→ 35-40
            4. **lactic acid: nml→ 35-50**
            5. methanol/ethanol: nml→ 35-50
    c. Non - Anion Gap metabolic acidosis (hyperchloremic)
        i.   Diarrhea
        ii. Renal tubular acidosis
        iii. Renal failure

3. Potassium: [K] helps to understand the patient's differential diagnosis
    a. Sources of potassium abnormality
        i.   Lab error (i.e., lysis of RBC in sample)
        ii. External gains (i.e. renal failure)
        iii. Transcellular shift (intracellular [K] = 150 mEq/l, extracellular [K] = 3.5)

b. Ddx of Hyperkalemia; ↑ [K]
    i. Acidosis: acidemia (high [H^+]) causes hyperkalemia by the H^+/K^+ exchanger in the cell membrane; H^+ moves from extracellular to intracellular, while K^+ is exchanged to the extracellular space (keeping the charge balanced).
    ii. HCO_3/Bicarbonate: when extracellular HCO_3 drops (is consumed via acidemia or leaves the body for some reason), HCO_3^- exits cells and K^+ follows; thus causing hyperkalemia.
    iii. Organic vs. inorganic acids causing a ↑ [K]:
       1. inorganic acids: ↑↑↑↑↑ [K]; non - anion gap metabolic acidosis (hyperchloremic) very, very, very much shifts K out of cells.
       2. organic acids: ↑ [K]; *lactic acid* has little effect on shifting K out of cells.
    iv. Insulin: low blood insulin levels cause K to come out of cells and glucose is usually high.
c. Ddx hypokalemia; ↓ [K]
    i. Alkalosis
    ii. Insulin: Insulin is given to patients with hyperkalemia to shift K into cells. Too much insulin given can cause hypokalemia, hypoglycemia and the patient can become unconscious (with hypoglycemia).

(ABG) Arterial Blood Gas

pH   / PaCO$_2$ / PaO$_2$ / HCO$_3$ / O$_2$Sat / Base Excess +2
7.35-7.45 / 35-45 / 80-100 / 21-27 / 95-98 / #
        / mmHg / mmHg / mEq/L / % /

Note: The ABG is used to determine acid-base status as well as respiratory function.

The systematic approach:
1. pH. acidosis or alkalosis?
2. What is the primary disorder? respiratory/metabolic.
3. Is respiratory disturbance acute or chronic? Or a mixture?
4. For metabolic disturbances, is there adequate compensation?

The systematic approach:
1. pH. acidosis or alkalosis?
    Acidosis if pH is below 7.35
    Alkalosis if pH is above 7.45

2. What is the primary disorder?
    Acidosis
        PaCO$_2$: if above 45 then primary respiratory acidosis
        HCO$_3$: if below 21 then primary metabolic acidosis
        Mixed disorder: if both are true
    Alkalosis
        PaCO$_2$: if below 35 then primary respiratory alkalosis
        HCO$_3$: if above 27 then primary metabolic alkalosis
        Mixed disorder: if both are true

3. Is respiratory disturbance acute or chronic? Or a mixture? The purpose of this is to help determine ventilation settings (i.e., what is the pt's baseline PaCO$_2$?)

Respiratory acidosis:
Acute: HCO$_{3expected}$ = a rise of 1 mEq/l in HCO$_3$ above baseline, for each 10mmHg rise in PaCO$_2$.
Chronic: HCO$_{3expected}$ = a rise of 4 mEq/l in HCO$_3$ above baseline, for each 10mmHg rise in PaCO$_2$.
acidosis mix of acute & chronic: HCO$_{3expected(acute)}$ < pt's HCO$_3$ < HCO$_{3expected(chronic)}$

Respiratory alkalosis:
Acute: HCO$_{3expected}$ = a decrease of 2 mEq/l in HCO$_3$ below baseline for each 10mmHg drop in PaCO$_2$.
Chronic: HCO$_{3expected}$ = a decrease of 5 mEq/l in HCO$_3$ below baseline for each 10mmHg drop in PaCO$_2$.
alkalosis mix of acute & chronic: HCO$_{3expected(acute)}$ > pt's HCO$_3$ > HCO$_{3expected(chronic)}$

If Pt's HCO$_3$ = HCO$_{3expected}$ ($\pm$2): buffering and renal systems are compensating properly

71

4. For metabolic disturbances, is the respiratory system adequately compensating?

Winter's formula: $PaCO_{2expected} = 1.5(HCO_3) + (8\pm2)$

Metabolic acidosis: $PaCO_{2expected}$ should follow Winter's formula
If Pt's $PaCO_2 = PaCO_{2expected}$ (±2): respiratory system is compensating properly
If Pt's $PaCO_2 > PaCO_{2expected}$ then a primary respiratory acidosis also exists
If Pt's $PaCO_2 < PaCO_{2expected}$ then a primary respiratory alkalosis also exists

Metabolic alkalosis: $PaCO_{2expected}$ should be a rise of 1-0.5mmHg in $PaCO_2$ for each 1 mEq/l rise in HCO_3 above baseline.
 (this doesn't follow Winter's formula exactly; should be about 40-50mmHg)
If Pt's $PaCO_2 = PaCO_{2expected}$ (±2):respiratory system is compensating properly
If Pt's $PaCO_2 > PaCO_{2expected}$ then a primary respiratory acidosis also exists
If Pt's $PaCO_2 < PaCO_{2expected}$ then a primary respiratory alkalosis also exists

Differential diagnoses for various disorders
Metabolic Acidosis
 Non-anion gap: GI HCO_3 loss (diarrhea, ureteral diversion, lower GI fistula), Renal HCO_3 loss (renal tubular acidosis, renal failure, carbonic anhydrase inhibitors), HCl administration, post hypocapnia

 Anion gap: (MUDPILES) Methanol, Uremia (renal failure- Rhabdomyolysis), DKA, Paraldehydes, Isoniazide, *Lactic acidosis* (hypoxemia, shock, CO, cyanide, hepatic failure, methemoglobinemia), Ethanol/ethylene glycol, Salicylates

Metabolic Alkalosis
Vomiting, NG tube suction/ upper GI fistula, diuretics (thiazide & loop), post hypercapnia (recovery in COPD), excess mineralocorticoids (aldosterone- Conn syndrome) or excess glucocorticoids (cortisol/steroids – Cushing syndrome), licorice ingestion, increased rennin states, Bartter's syn, excess alkali administration, refeeding alkalosis

Respiratory Acidosis
 Acute: CNS depression (drugs/stroke), myopathies, neuropathies, acute airway obstruction, pneumonia (late), pulmonary edema (late), impaired lung motion (PTX, hemothorax), flail chest, late/large pulmonary embolus, ventilator dysfunction

 Chronic: COPD, restrictive lung disease, chronic neuromuscular disorders, chronic respiratory center depression

Respiratory Alkalosis, acute
anxiety, hypoxia (asthma, pneumonia), lung or CNS disease, drugs (salicylates, catecholamines, progesterone), pregnancy, pulmonary embolus (early/mild), sepsis (early shock), hepatic encephalopathy, mechanical ventilation (over ventilating)

Examples Cases:
1. Na 123, K 5.9, Cl 86, HCO$_3$ 9, BUN 81, Cr 2.3, Gluc 361, Ca 8.5, Phos 6.5.
This is a 45yo morbidly obese male who came into the ER with a HR of 145, BP 90/50 with the above labs and complaining of fatigue & SOB. These labs should make you think something serious is going on. Note the low HCO$_3$ in conjunction with a K which is mildly elevated-means lactic acid. An ABG (with a lactic acid) and an EKG should also be ordered. Erythema was on his inner left thigh. Answer: necrotizing fascitis; his heart rate was fast from the acidosis (lactic) and hypotension from septic shock. Patient's chance of survival is inversely related to the time from onset of fascitis to OR debridement. This patient died.

2. Admission: Na 132, K 4.4, Cl 98, HCO$_3$ 23, BUN 122, Cr 6.8(3.4 base line), Gluc 183, Ca 8.5, Mg 2.1 Phos 6.3, WBC 12.5, H/H 12/36, PLT 172.
73y M s/p cardiac cath developing dye associated renal failure, 6 days later developed pneumonia, placed on Avelox and Zithromax, dc'd from hospital 10 day ago now in ER with +N +V diarrhea. Cardiac cath showed severe Pulmonary HTN 88/38 and severe LV dysfunction. Vitals stable, admitted to floor, C.Diff toxin sent, empirically treated for C. Diff. Next day lethargy and hypotensive, transferred to MICU.
Na 130, K 4.7, Cl 97, HCO$_3$ 19, BUN 122, Cr 6.0, Gluc 248 ABG 7.28/36/79/17/-9
ABG 7.28/36/79/17/-9; lactic acid 2.4
Notice the gap acidosis & elevated, but low potassium and how this is predictive of the lactic acid level. Lactic acid is indicative of dying tissue. This patient died.

3. Na 123 Cl 99 pH 7.31 PaCO$_2$ 10 HCO$_3$ 5
Answer: anion gap metabolic acidosis, primary respiratory alkalosis and non-anion gap metabolic acidosis

4. Na 130 Cl 80 pH 7.20 PaCO$_2$ 25 HCO$_3$ 10
Answer: anion gap metabolic acidosis with primary metabolic alkalosis
Clinical: Diabetic pt with viral gastroenteritis, nausea & vomiting resulting in volume loss, hypokalemia=>metabolic alkalosis. Pt stops taking insulin, resulting in DKA

5. Na 125 Cl 100 K 2.5 pH 7.07 PaCO$_2$ 28 HCO$_3$ 8
Answer: anion gap metabolic acidosis, non anion gap metabolic acidosis & respiratory acidosis Clinical: Respiratory acidosis most likely from secondary muscle weakness secondary to hypokalemia. (hypokalemia with acidosis is going to require a ton of total body K to be replaced). If giving HCO$_3$ would push K into cells and endanger respirations even more & possible precipitate respiratory or cardiac arrest. So respiratory support with mechanical ventilation should be done first before correcting the acidosis and hypokalemia.

References
Abelow, B. Understanding Acid-Base Williams & Wilkins, Baltimore, 1998.
Haber, RJ. *A Practical Approach to Aid-Base Disorders.* The Western Journal of Medicine 1991; 155(2):146-151.

Notes

Clinical Nutrition/Electrolytes

Why is nutrition clinically important?
The body can not heal without the proper building blocks. Organ systems respond differently to stress/sickness when a patient is malnourished. In order to understand a patient's condition and institute a treatment plan which will work successfully, both in the acute and long term phase, you must understand how malnourishment will affect your treatment plan. The immune system and wound healing are highly dependent upon the ability to make protein in order to accomplish their missions; malnourishment severely affects these ends. The malnourished sick patient has a reduced ability to respond to stress. There is a 2-3 fold increased loss of protein in the stressed sick patient. This protein loss can be slowed by adding dextrose. The goal of nutritional support is to provide amino acids via protein to optimize protein synthesis. If protein can not be given, then to minimize protein losses, give carbohydrates. Albumin <3.5 means there is a severe problem (malnutrition); 2.5 means that 2/3 of the total body albumin is gone. Operative mortality is 20 fold higher in malnourished patients.

A clinical example is the surgeon who is asked to place a gastrostomy tube (a feeding tube into the stomach which exits the abdominal wall). There are usually two choices, a percutaneous endoscopic gastrostomy (PEG) or an open gastrostomy tube. The PEG has several advantages of being fast and minimally invasive to the patient but requires the stomach to adhere (via scar tissue) the abdominal wall. The open technique requires a midline incision, where the abdominal contents are visualized and the stomach is actually sutured to the abdominal wall (around the gastrostomy tube. In the scenario where the patient is malnourished the open technique is probably a better choice as the sutures will hold the stomach in place while the body scars the stomach to the abdominal wall, around the tube. The PEG procedure would risk the stomach falling away from the abdominal wall creating the equivalent of an abdominal organ perforation, which the patient could died from if not repaired emergently.

Systematic approach
1. Which patients need nutrition support? Which route is optimal for support?
   Contraindications/risks.
3. What are the nutritional requirements/design a formula?
4. Start, monitor, and evaluate/change therapy.

1. **Which patients need support/Route/ Contraindications/Risks:**
   a. General: Who needs support? (Most do not.)
      i. If NPO for 5 days, start.
      ii. If the patient will not be eating anytime soon, then start nutritional support immediately.
      iii. The malnourished/catabolic patient.
         1. Lab tests:
            a. Serum albumin: <3.5 g/dL (half life: 14-20 days)
            b. Serum prealbumin: 10-15 mild depletion
                              5-10   moderate depletion
                              <5   severe depletion (half life: 2-3 days)
            c. Serum tansferrin: <200 mg/dL (half life 8-10 days)

        iv.   Immune function derangement.
               a.   ABS Lymphocyte count 1,500 – 1800 mild
                               900 – 1500 moderate
                               <900 severe depletion
        v.   Excessive protein losses.
               1.   GI tract fistula
               2.   Ileostomy
               3.   Draining gastrostomy
               4.   Burns
               5.   Seeping wounds

b.   Protein Sparing:
        i.   Short term for well nourished patients (not for malnourished/stressed patients)
        ii.   100g of dextrose a day can spare protein (2L D5 or 2L D5NS or 1L D10)

c.   Oral or Tube Feeds (Enteral Support):
        i.   General: If the GI tract (or a part of it) is able to absorb nutrients, then as a general rule try that route first. Intestinal epithelium acts as a barrier to bacterial translocation into the blood. Bowel rest causes atrophy of the epithelium; enteral feeding prevents this atrophy. Using the GI tract is usually in the patient's best interest. Tube feeds are for patients which have a functional GI tract, but are unable to take food orally.
        ii.   Requirements: Need bowel function (need all three, stomach/small bowel/colon to function).
               1.   Small bowel: +BS: Small bowel usually has some function, even several hrs post op, but the stomach and colon may not. The stomach and duodenum are usually the last to start working (thus they may be bypassed). –BS – Flatus can usually still handle tube feeds OK. If distended and tender belly stop tube feeds.
               2.   Stomach: NGT output low means gastric function. This doesn't imply that the bowel is functioning.
               3.   Colon: +BM and +Flatus means the colon is working. This doesn't necessarily imply that the bowel is functioning.
        iii.   Contraindications:
               1.   Circulatory shock
               2.   Intestinal ischemia
               3.   Enterocolitis
               4.   Bowel obstruction
               5.   Ileus
               6.   GI bleed
               7.   Vomiting
        iv.   Not advised
               1.   Severe diarrhea
               2.   Pancreatitis (partial enteral nutrition is OK if in jejunum)
               3.   Fistula >500ml per day

d.   TPN:
        i.   Usually used only if tube feeds are not possible secondary to the gut not working.
        ii.   Requirements: Central line (Hickman catheter) or PICC (peripherally inserted central catheter) line

iii. TPN Complications:
1. Central line problems: PTX, infection, etc.
2. Hyperglycemia:
   a. 30% of insulin adsorbs to the tubes and bag
   b. When TPN is stopped the insulin requirement will be less
3. Hypophosphatemia: glucose entry into cells causes ↓PO4 (and the manufacture of ATP). Refeeding syndrome is the extreme of this where there isn't enough ATP to breath.
4. Hypernatremia. Precipitation of CHF.
5. Fatty liver: if glucose>daily requirement, lipogenesis in the liver (↑ LFTs)
6. Hypercapnia: excessive carbohydrates & over feeding in general
7. Oxidant injury: lipid infusions cause oxidant induced cell injury (free fatty acids are known to cause pulmonary capillary damage and ARDS
8. Bowel atrophy: translocation & septicemia
9. Acalculus cholecystitis: bile stasis (eventual rupture of gallbladder if not treated)

e. PPN: peripheral parenteral nutrition is also possible (about 12% dextrose)
  i. No need for a central line (peripheral IV is adequate)
  ii. A solution <950 mosm/L to prevent vein phlebitis
  iii. Hypocaloric (not complete nutrition)
  iv. Large volume of solution
  v. Example of a typical 'emergency bag' of 1L PPN: 950mosm/L

Protein:	50g	Dextrose:	200 Kcal	Lipid:	400 Kcal
Sodium:	37 mEq	Chloride:	30 mEq	Acetate:	35 mEq
Phosphate:	9 mEq	Calcium:	5 mEq	Magnesium:	5 mEq
+ Trace elements and multivitamin					

2. **Requirements**
a. Total energy
  i. BMR (basal metabolic rate)
   1. estimated by Harris-Benedict eqn (see end of section)
      a. BMR Men = 66+(13.75*wt)+(5*ht)-(6.8*age)
      b. BMR Women = 655+(9.56*wt)+(1.85*ht)-(4.68*age)
      c. use ideal weights, not actual weights
      d. wt[kg] (note: obese wt=ideal*1.3); ht=[cm]; age=[yrs]
   2. Quick estimation: **BMR =25-35 kcal/kg/day**
  ii. Adjustments to BMR (multiply by one of the highest applicable numbers)
   1. Burn injury   2.1
   2. Trauma with steroids   1.8
   3. Major sepsis   1.6
   4. Temp>38 & Minute ventilation>200ml/kg/min   1.65
   5. Liver Failure   1.5
   6. Pancreatitis   1.5
   7. Temp>38 or Minute ventilation>200ml/kg/min   1.4
   8. Acute Renal Failure   1.3
   9. Skeletal trauma   1.35
   10. Peritonitis   1.25
   11. Minor trauma   1.2
   12. Post op   1.05

b. Protein requirement (ideal body weights) (4 kcal/g):
   i. Normal: 0.8-1.0 g/kg (albumin >3.5)
   ii. Moderate malnutrition: 1.5g/kg (albumin 2.8-3.5)
   iii. Marked malnutrition 2.0g/kg (albumin <2.8)
   iv. Daily Protein turnover: 300g (about 3% of total body protein)

c. Carbohydrates (ideal body weights) (4 kcal/g):
   i. Total non protein calories 10-40 Kcal/kg/day (usually 40-100% of total non protein calories)
   ii. Maximum: 7g/kg/day

d. Lipids (ideal body weights) (9 kcal/g):
   i. Total non protein calories 10-40 Kcal/kg/day (usually 0-60% of total non protein calories)
   ii. Maximum: <0.5-1.0g/kg/day
   iii. Not in TPN for 1wk for patients on Propofol, severely injured or septic.

3. **TPN – design a nutritional support formula**
  a. 2 methods: Every hospital perform this a different way (you have to know both methods)
   i. 1st method: Pharmacy does most of the work
   ii. 2nd method: Physician has to select and modify formula for specific needs.

  b. 1st Method: pharmacy does most of the work
   i. **Energy**: BMR * stress factor = total kcal needed in formula

   ii. **Protein** (4.0 kcal/g): # g/day
     1. usually 1.5g/kg
     2. hypercatabolism 1.2-1.6 g/kg
     3. 1yr olds: 2g/kg
     4. range 0.5-2.5 g/kg
     5. Volume in a protein bag: 10ml/g protein (some solns are less)
   iii. **Non-protein calories = Energy – protein kcal**

   iv. **Non-protein calories (carbohydrates + lipids)**: #kcal/day
     1. Total non protein calories 10-40 Kcal/kg
     2. Non protein calories usually 25 Kcal/kg
     3. Volume, minimal: 0.5 ml/Kcal
     4. **Dextrose** (3.4 kcal/g): #kcal/day
       a. start lower and increase over days
       b. usu 65% of non-protein calories
     5. **Lipids** (9.1 kcal/g): #kcal/day
       a. usu 35% of non-protein calories
       b. If the patient is on Propofol, don't give lipids

   v. **Total Volume**: ml/day (protein vol + non-protein vol + 100ml (electrolytes/additives))
     Volume = 10ml/g protein + 0.5 ml/Kcal non protein Kcal +100ml

   vi. **Electrolytes:** These are adjusted by the patient's chem-7
     1. **Sodium** 60-100 mEq/day (sodium acetate or sodium chloride)

a. Think about NS 154mEq/l; 1/2NS 77mEq/l
b. Too rapid correction of hyponatremia can case central pontine myelinolysis.
2. **Potassium** 50-90 mEq/day (potassium chloride or potassium acetate)
   a. Start with 1-1.5mEq/kg; adjust based upon the previous 24hrs
   b. Renal failure: usually don't give K
3. **Chloride/Acetate**
   a. Adjusted by the patient's acid/base status
   b. Add acetate if:
      i. Lung and kidney are not working normally
      ii. Acid losses: NGT output
      iii. Base losses: fistula, ileostomy, diarrhea
      iv. Low $HCO3$; also don't try to 'fix' $HCO3$ (for compensating for altered $pCO2$) with TPN.
4. **Phosphorous** 20-50 mmol/day (sodium phosphate or potassium phosphate)
   a. Start with 20mmol/day; adjust based upon the previous 24hrs
   b. Renal failure: usu don't give PO4
   c. 1 mmol KPO4 = 1.47 mEq K; 1 mmol NaPO4 = 1.33 mEq Na
5. **Calcium** 10-22 mEq/day (calcium gluconate)
   a. Start with 15mEq/day
   b. Note: ensure (PO4*2/TPN vol)+(Ca/TPN vol) <= 60 (so it doesn't precipitate in solution)
6. **Magnesium** 15-30 mEq/day (magnesium sulfate)
   a. Start with 25mEq/day
   b. 8 mEq Mg = 1g MgSO4
   c. Renal failure: usu don't give Mg
7. **Other additions:**
   a. Multivitamin.
      i. Vit K is not in this.
      ii. Vit K, C and zinc are important for wound healing.
   b. Insulin
      i. Sub Q first. To determine a patinet's needs then usu give 2/3rds of the total via TPN bag.
      ii. 1/3 of the total insulin injected into the bag usu adheres to the plastic tubing and never makes it to the patient.
   c. Heparin
   d. Vit K 10mg q wk (unless the patient is on Warfarin)
   e. Trace elements
      i. Copper
      ii. Chromium
      iii. Manganese
      iv. Selenium
      v. Zinc
   f. H2 blockers

c. 2nd Method: Physician has to select and modify formula for specific needs.
  i. Physician has to select and modify formula for specific needs.
  ii. Modified example taken from Marino, <u>The ICU Book</u>
    1. Estimate the protein and calorie requirements (see above).
    2. Determine the volume of 10%AA-50% dextrose solution needed to deliver the protein requirements (really it's a 5%AA-25%dextrose solution as 50g AA/1 L + 250g dextrose/L).
      a. Other available standard solutions can be determined using the same example:
        i. Low Protein: 12%AA/65%Dex/23%Fat (30gAA/191gDex/26gFat)
        ii. Intermediate Protein 16%AA/60%Dex/24%Fat (40gAA/176gDex/27gFat)
        iii. etc.
    3. Determine the number of calories delivered by the above AA/dex solution.
    4. Using the 10% lipid emulsion soln, determine the amount needed to account for the difference needed in calories (max rate of 50ml/hr of lipid). Example (all based on one day) :

    Calories: 30 kcal/kg * 70 kg * 1.2 stress = 2520 kcal/day
    Protein: 1.4 g/kg * 70 kg = 98 g protein
    98g * 1L/50g AA = 1.9 L (81 ml/hr)
    1.9L * 250g dex/1 L = 475g * 3.4 kcal/1g dex = 1615 kcal
    1.9L * 50g protein/1 L = 95 g * 4.0 kcal/1g = 380 kcal
    2520 kcal - 1615 kcal – 380 kcal = 525 kcal for lipid
    525 kcal * 1ml/ 1kcal 10% lipid = 525 ml (round, 500 ml over 12 hrs)

d. Standard formula
  i. Usually TPN is ordered before noon, as some hospitals have to send away for the formulation to be made. If a patient needs a bag after that time a 'standard bag' or 'emergency bag' is ordered. Or D10W can be given.
  ii. It would be poor form to continually give a patient the standard bag when you could custom tailor it for their clinical scenario.
  iii. Example of a typical 'emergency bag' of TPN 1L:

Protein: 50g   Dextrose: 600 Kcal   Lipid: 250 Kcal
Sodium: 37 mEq   Chloride: 30 mEq   Acetate: 35 mEq
Phosphate: 9 mEq Calcium: 5 mEq   Magnesium:5 mEq
+ Trace elements and multivitamin

e. Initiation of TPN: start at 1000 kcal and increase by 500 kcal/day.

f. Stopping: When the patient can take 75% of his calories enterally.

4. **Tube feeds - design a nutritional support formula**
  a. Select a formula
    i. Polymeric vs. Monomeric
      1. Polymeric, Peptide based formula (not predigested, food in can):
        a. Free AA, dipeptides & tripeptides
        b. Fatty Acids: medium chain
        c. Carbs: maltodextran

2. Monomeric, Elemental based formula (predigested)
   a. Jejunal feeds in patients with pancreatitis
   b. For patients with impaired digestive absorption
   c. Free AA
   d. No fatty acids
   e. Carbs: maltodextran

   ii. Caloric density: 1-1.5 kcal/ml or 2.0 kcal/ml (for Volume restricted pts)
   iii. Osm: [280-1100mOsm/kg water] (hypertonic solns should be infused into stomach to prevent diarrhea & abdominal pain- as opposed to jejunum)
   iv. Protein: usu 35-40g/l (formulas designated HN mean 'high nitrogen', more protein, 60g/l)
   v. Lipids: 30% in most feeds

b. Usual diets:
   i. Std surgical: isosource, Ensure
   ii. Renal: Ensure Plus, nutren 2.0 (limits elec., fluid & protein; 2 Kcal/ml (lower feed rates))
   iii. Ex: For a 70 kg person, 25kcal/kg, 1750 ml Isosource or 875 ml Nutren 2.0 (36ml/hr)

c. Specific diets: CHF, renal, hepatic, pulmonary, critical care, immunosuppression
   i. For patients in respiratory failure: Pulmocare: 55% lipids (to decrease CO_2)
   ii. For patients with inflammation mediated tissue injury:
       1. Impact: fishoils & arginine (to improve immune fxn)
       2. Perative: fishoils & Beta carotene (antioxidant)

d. Additives
   i. Alitra Q: provides 0.35/kg/day of glutamine, the primary fuel for the bowel mucosa (all formulas have it to a lesser extent)
   ii. Fiber: helps to prevent translocation
   iii. TraumaAid & Stresstein: for trauma patients
   iv. HepaticAidII & Travasorb hepatic: for hepatic encephalopathic patients
   v. Glucerna, Isocal HN, Jevity, Peptamen: all contain elevated levels of carnitine; deficiencies can occur in prolonged hypercatabolic states
   vi. Elemental diets: good for fistulas, IBD, post op ileus, colonic fistula, short bowel syndrome, radiation enteritis, pancreatitis, decubitus ulcers.

e. Starting a regiment.
   i. Tube types: (post pyloric tubes are always preferred to reduce the aspiration risk)
       a. Nasogastric (NGT)
       b. Nasojejunal (e.g., Keofeed, Dobhoff)
       c. Gastrostomy (G-Tube, PEG) (see section intro)
       d. Jejunostomy (J-tube)
   ii. Ensure tube is correctly placed in the bowel (not lungs via CXR/KUB)
       1. Gastric feeds (bolus feeds):
           i. Start: 50-100 ml every 4 hrs. increase by 50ml to goal.
           ii. First bolus: Infuse water, clamp tube, wait 30 min, aspirate residual volume.

     iii. Before each bolus: aspirate gastric contents 'Gastric residuals' to ensure fluid is not accumulating. If the volume is half or greater than the infused amount, then hold the next bolus.

     iv. After the bolus: flush the tube with 30ml water.

1. If vol is <50% of infused volume, proceed with planned feeds
2. If vol is >50% of infused volume, think about duodenal/jejunal feeds or not ready for feeds yet.

2. Postpyloric feeds (continuous feeds):
   a. Use starter regiment
   b. Ex. Start 20ml/hr for first 8 hrs, then increase by 10 - 20ml/hr every 4 - 8hrs until goal feed rate is reached. Water flushes 30 ml every 4 hrs.
   c. Feed for 12-15 hrs then rest for 12-8 hrs (anything more can cause bowel stress and diarrhea)

f.   Tube feed complications.
  i.   Feeds not moving through: abdominal distention or pain should be indications to slow or stop.
  ii.   Tube occlusion:
      1. Prevention: 30ml of water flush Q4hrs & 10 ml flush after meds
      2. Relieve obstruction:
         a. Warm water with syringe irrigation.
         b. Flush with soda or pancreatic enzymes ('Declogger')
  iii. Aspiration:
         a. Decrease risk, elevate the head of bed 30 deg.
         b. High gastric residuals. Try Reglan or erythromycin
  iv. Diarrhea
      1. C.diff is often a concern if a patient develops diarrhea.
      2. Fat infused past the duodenum will cause diarrhea.
      3. Lactose in a lactose-intolerant patient.
  v.   Hypoprothrombinemia: Vit K deficiency (bleeding)
  vi. Dehydration: bolus tap water 200-300 ml Q4-8hrs.
  vii. Hyperosmolarity: hypernatremia.
  viii. Hyperglycemia.

5. **Monitoring**
   a. Vitals: Q6 hrs
   b. Glucose: Q6hrs until normal then Daily; If glucose>200 then decrease the carbs or add insulin to TPN bag.
   c. Weight: Daily
   d. Electrolytes:
     i.   Daily: Chem-7 panel + Mg + PO4 + Ca (until normal then 3x Qwk)
     ii.   Weekly: LFTs, CBC, PT/INR, bilirubin, triglycerides
   e. Protein:
     i.   After 3 days get a '24hr urine for urea nitrogen' (UUN)
     ii.   Nitrogen balance = protein intake (#g last 24hrs)/6.25 – UUN (#g last 24hrs) + 4g (daily nitrogen losses) [Note: 16% of protein is nitrogen or 1g nitrogen/6.25g of protein; UUN is urine urea nitrogen; if UUN>30 then daily losses should be 6, not 4]
     iii. Goal: to maintain a positive balance of 4-6 grams

Electrolyte replacement (ad lib replacement)

Better to replace PO if possible; IV is necessary often (rapid correction or the patient is NPO to everything, i.e. a fresh proximal anastomosis). All values are for adults, unless otherwise specified.

Hypomagnesemia [normal 1.6 - 2.6] (replacement can cause hypotension; HD can't decrease Mg levels in the body)
Most frequent order: 1-2g $MgSO_4$ IV x 1

Mild:[<1.5 mEq/L] *Magnesium Oxide 1g PO QD* (may cause diarrhea)
Mod:[<1.0 asymptomatic] *Magnesium Sulfate 1g/hr IV for 3-4 hr* (DTR & levels)
Severe:[<1.0 symptomatic] *Magnesium Sulfate 2g in D_5W IV over 10-20 min* then *1 g/hr for 3-4 hrs* (follow DTRs & Mg levels)
($\downarrow$Mg can cause $\downarrow$Ca & hyperactive DTRs; usu also $\downarrow$K and $\downarrow PO_4$ exist)

Hypophosphatemia [Adults 2.5–4.5; Kids 4.0-6.0] (usually not given to HD patients. Also given to prevent refeeding syndrome)
Most frequent order: 10 - 20 mmole KPO_4 IV x 1

Mild/Mod:[>1.5 mg/dL] $NaPO_4$(*Neutra-Phos*) or KPO_4(*K-Phos*) *1-2 tablets PO BID or TID* (250-500 mg PO_4 or 8mM/tablet)
$NaPO_4$(*Fleet's Phospho-soda*) *5mL PO BID or TID* (128 mg PO_4 or 4mM/mL)
Severe:[<1.0-1.5 symptomatic] **(rapid correction can precipitate $\downarrow$Ca**; PO preferred)
$NaPO_4$ or KPO_4 2mg/kg (0.08mM/kg) IV over 6hrs

Hypokalemia [3.5 – 5 mEq/L] (what is the renal status? Check before replacement)
Most frequent order: 10-20 mEq KCl IV x 1 then recheck K level.

Usually: [K] 2.0 = a deficit of 200 mEq/L (70kg adult)
      To change from 3 to 4 takes about 100 mEq/L of potassium (70kg adult)
Treat underlying cause for hypokalemia?
Digoxin? If so treat $\downarrow$K aggressively. Treat $\downarrow$Mg if present.
Slow correction: KCl via PO

Powder	K-Lor	KCl	15 or 20 mEq/packet
Liquid	Kaochlor 10%	KCl	20mEq/15ml
Liquid	Kaon-Cl 20%	KCl	40mEq/15ml
Liquid	Kaon elixir	Gluconate	20mEq/mL
Tabs (large in size)	Tabs-slow release also avail.		
Adults: 20-40 mEq PO BID or TID	Peds: 1-2 mEq/kg/d divided doses		

Rapid correction: replacement via 10-20 mEq IV KCl x 1 then recheck K level (Heart monitor if >20 mEq/hr IV) (can replace Maximum:40 mEq IV KCL x 1 after much experience)

Peds: <40 kg: 0.25 mEq/kg/hr x 2hrs; >40 kg: 16-20 mEq/hr x 2hr
severe [<2 mEq/L] 20-40 mEq/hr IV (recheck K level every 1- 2 hrs)

Calcium [8.4 – 10.2 mEq/L]
Most frequent order: 1g CaCl IV x 1

Usually Ca is false low secondary to low albumin and is not replaced; so you must check the corrected level: Ca corrected = Ca + 0.8(4 – [albumin])

However, if the patient is bleeding and being given blood (which has citrate in it to prevent the blood from clotting), then calcium is usually given to reverse the anticoagulation citrate effects and help stop bleeding (calcium is a cofactor of many coagulation proteins).

Nutrition card

Protein req. (ideal weights)		Albumin
Normal: 0.8-1.0 g/kg		>3.5
Mod. malnutrition: 1.5g/kg		2.8-3.5
Marked malnutrition 2.0g/kg		<2.8

Harris-Benedict eqns
Total Energy Requirments   adjustment [1.2]   Std calc 25-35kcal/kg/day

Men

Height	ideal weight lbs	kg	BMR	10	20	30	40	50	60	70	80	90	25	30	35	Protein g/kg/day 1.0	1.5	2.0	Protein Kcal/day 1.0	1.5	2.0
5' 0"	120	54	152	1810	1728	1647	1565	1484	1402	1320	1239	1157	1361	1633	1905	54	82	109	218	327	43
5' 2"	130	59	157	1915	1834	1752	1670	1589	1507	1426	1344	1262	1474	1769	2063	59	88	118	236	354	47
5' 4"	140	63	163	2021	1939	1857	1776	1694	1613	1531	1449	1368	1587	1905	2222	63	95	127	254	381	50
5' 6"	150	68	168	2126	2044	1963	1881	1799	1718	1636	1555	1473	1701	2041	2381	68	102	136	272	408	54
5' 8"	160	73	173	2231	2150	2068	1986	1905	1823	1742	1660	1578	1814	2177	2540	73	109	145	290	435	58
5' 10"	170	77	178	2337	2255	2173	2092	2010	1929	1847	1765	1684	1927	2313	2698	77	116	154	308	463	61
6' 0"	180	82	183		2360	2279	2197	2115	2034	1952	1871	1789	2041	2449	2857	82	122	163	327	490	65
6' 2"	190	86	188		2466	2384	2302	2221	2139	2058	1976	1894	2154	2585	3016	86	129	172	345	517	68
6' 4"	200	91	193		2571	2489	2408	2326	2244	2163	2081	2000	2268	2721	3175	91	136	181	363	544	72

Women

Height	ideal weight lbs	kg	BMR	10	20	30	40	50	60	70	80	90	25	30	35
5' 0"	120	54	152	1692	1636	1580	1524	1468	1412	1356	1299	1243	1361	1633	1905
5' 2"	130	59	157	1756	1700	1643	1587	1531	1475	1419	1363	1307	1474	1769	2063
5' 4"	140	63	163	1819	1763	1707	1651	1594	1538	1482	1426	1370	1587	1905	2222
5' 6"	150	68	168	1882	1826	1770	1714	1658	1602	1545	1489	1433	1701	2041	2381
5' 8"	160	73	173	1946	1890	1833	1777	1721	1665	1609	1553	1496	1814	2177	2540
5' 10"	170	77	178	2009	1953	1897	1841	1784	1728	1672	1616	1560	1927	2313	2698
6' 0"	180	82	183		2016	1960	1904	1848	1792	1735	1679	1623	2041	2449	2857
6' 2"	190	86	188		2079	2023	1967	1911	1855	1799	1743	1686	2154	2585	3016
6' 4"	200	91	193		2143	2087	2030	1974	1918	1862	1806	1750	2268	2721	3175

Adjustments to total energy
(multiply BMR by the highest applicable numb...)

Burn injury	2.1
Trauma with steroids	1.8
Trauma	1.6
Major sepsis	1.6
T>38 & Minute vent >200ml/kg/min	1.65
T>38 or Minute vent >200ml/kg/min	1.4
Skeletal trauma	1.35
Peritonitis	1.25
Minor trauma	1.2
Post op	1.05

References:
Paul L. Marino, The ICU Book, 2nd ed.
David Frankenfield, Penn State, Dept. of Surgery Handbook, 7th ed., 2004
Carlos Pestana, Fluids and Electrolytes in the Surgical Patient, 5th ed., 2000
The Washington Manual of Surgery, 4th ed., 2005

Tough Words

Some of these words you many know, but you may not be able to define if someone asked you. Remember, words have specific meaning and some people become very upset when you use words incorrectly (especially when presenting during rounds). I made this list of words I found myself having to lookup multiple times during M3 & M4 years. These definitions came form Taber's cyclopedic medical dictionary, 18th edition.

Adenitis – inflammation of lymph nodes or a gland.

Adnexal – adjacent or appending.

Ameliorate – to make better or more tolerable; to grow better.

Anasarca – severe generalized edema.

Anergia – inactivity; lack of energy (e.g., HIV pts exhibit anergy when given a PPD test).

Anhedonia – lack of pleasure in acts that are normally pleasurable.

Anhidrosis – diminished or complete absence of secretion of sweat.

Anosmia – loss of the sense of smell.

Apnea – temporary cessation of breathing.

Apposite – highly pertinent or appropriate.

Apropos – at the opportune time; being both relevant and opportune.

Canonical – conforming to a general rule or acceptable procedure: orthodox.

Catarrhal – inflammation of a mucus membrane esp. nose & air passages.

Cerclage – encircling tissues with a ligature, wire or loop.

Chadwick's sign – a deep blue-violet color of the cervix & vagina caused by increased vascularity; a presumptive sign that is evident around the 4th week of gestation.

Chalazion – small hard tumor analogous to a sebaccous cyst developing in eyelids, formed by distention of a meibomian gland with secretion.

Cheilitus – inflammation of the lip.

Chloasma – pigmentary skin discolorations usually in occurring yellowish-brown patches or spots (often occurs in pregnancy and then disappears after delivery).

Cinchonism – poisoning from cinchona or its alkaloids (quinidine) marked by temporary deafness, headache, vertigo, tinnitus and rash.

Claudication - calf pain only when walking.

Convalescence – the period of recovery after the termination of an disease or operation.

Coryza – an acute catarrhal inflammation of the nasal mucus membrane with profuse nasal discharge.

Defervesence – the period that marks the subsidence of fever to normal temperature.

Dehiscence – a bursting open of a wound, especially a surgical abdominal wound.

Delirium – a state of mental confusion & excitement marked by disorientation for time and place, usually with illusions and hallucinations. The mind wanders, speech is incoherent and the patient is in a state of continual aimless physical activity.

Delusion – something that is falsely believed or propagated.

Dermatographism – a form of physical allergy in which a pale raised wheal with red flare on each side is produced when the skin is scratched by using a blunt object.

Diaphoresis – profuse sweating.

Diathesis – a constitutional predisposition to certain disease conditions.

Dysarthria – 1. inability to speak in which there is no defect in the ability to understand, read, or write. 2. difficult and defective speech due to impairment of the tongue or other muscles essential to speech. Mental function is intact.

Dysdiadochokinesia – the inability to quickly substitute antagonistic motor impulses to produce antagonistic muscular movements.

Dysmenorrhea - pain upon menstruation.

Dysphoria- an exaggerated feeling of depression and unrest without apparent cause; a mood of general dissatisfaction, unpleasantness, restlessness & anxiety, discomfort and unhappiness.

Dyspareunia – pain in the labia, vagina, or pelvis during or after sexual intercourse.

Dyspraxia – a disturbance of programming, control and execution of volitional movements.

Dystaxia – partially defective muscular coordination, esp. that manifested when voluntary muscular movements are attempted.

Dystocia – difficult labor.

Dystonia – prolonged muscle contractions that may cause twisting and repetitive movements or abnormal posture. These movements may be in the form of rhythmic jerks.

Endemic – pertaining to a disease which occurs continuously or in expected cycles in a population (e.g., The flu, the common cold) contrast to epidemic.

Emaciation – a state of being lean.

Encopresis – constipation and fecal retention where watery contents by pass hard fecal masses.

Enuresis – involuntary discharge of urine after an age where bladder control should have been established.

Eponym – a name for anything adapted from a person of location.

Epistaxis – nosebleeds.

Epulis – nonpathological softening/swelling of the gums due to hyperemia in the midtrimester pregnancy & subsides after pregnancy/delivery.

Escutcheon – the pattern of pubic growth (different in males and females).

Euphoria – a felling of well being or elation.

Exophthalmos – abnormal protrusion of the eyeball.

Fasciculations – involuntary contraction or twitching of muscle fibers, visible under the skin.

Fastidious – concerning an organism that has precise nutritional & environmental requirements for growth and survival.

Fibrillations – quivering or spontaneous contraction of individual muscle fibers.

Fiduciary relation – when one person justifiable reposes confidence, faith & reliance in another whose aid, advice, or protection is sought in some manner; good conscience requires one to act at all times for the sole benefit & interest of another with loyalty to those interests (required by law for certain classes of persons).

Fulminant – having rapid & severe onset.

Gravida – a pregnant woman.

Hegar's sign – present in 2 or 3rd month of pregnancy. On bimanual exam, the lower part of the uterus is easily compressed between fingers in vagina & fingers on abdomen (fetus doesn't fill it at this stage).

Hirsutism – a condition characterized by excessive growth of hair or the presence of hair in unusual places, esp. in women.

Hysteresis – a retardation of the effect when forces acting upon a body are changed (e.g., when you turn a hot water faucet, from a closed position, to 50% and get temperature 1. You then continue to turn it to 100%. Now as you close it back down to 50% again, you get temperature 2. The faucet is said to have a hysteresis associated with it when temperature 1 dose not equal 2.)

Iatrogenic – an adverse condition induced in a patient through the effects of treatment by a physician.

Lavage – washing; esp. therapeutic washing of an organ.

Lightening – the descent of the presenting part of the fetus into the pelvis, usually occurs 2-3 weeks before the first stage of labor begins.

Malady – a dz of disorder of the animal body.

Meconium – first feces of a newborn infant (salts, bile, cells) greenish black, orderless & tarry; first appears with in 24 hours, lasts 3 days.

Menometrorrhagia – irregular or excessive menstral bleeding.

Menorrhagia – excessive but regular menstrual bleeding.

Metrorrhagia – irregular vaginal bleeding.

Mortality – the proportion of deaths to population.

Morbidity – the proportion of diseased to population.

Munchausen syndrome – a patient which practices self multilation & deception in order to feign illness; usually leave one hospital and arrive in another. Usually patients are seldom recognized in time to receive psychiatric diagnosis & therapy, which they need.

Munchausen syndrome by proxy – the fabrication of symptoms or physical evidence of another's illness, or the deliberate causing of anothers' illness, to gain medical attention.

Mydriasis – abnormal dilation of the pupil.

Myoclonus – twitching or clonic spasm of a muscle or group of muscles.

Nidus – 1. a nest of breeding place especially a place in an animal or plant where bacteria lodge and multiply. 2. a place where something originates, develops or is located.

Nosocomial – Pertinent to or occurring in a hospital.

Nymphomania - excessive or abnormal sexual craving in the female (see satyriasis).

Odynophagia - pain upon swallowing.

Orthodeoxia – decreased oxygen concentration while upright (assoc. w/ infection of PCP or hepatopulmonary syn).

Orthopena – SOB in any position except an erect position.

Osteomalacia – a dz marked by increasing softness of the bones, so that they become flexible & brittle, thus causing deformities (adult form of rickets).

Palliative – to reduce the effect or intensity especially of a disease without curing.

Para – a woman who has produced a viable infant (>500g or >20 wk gestation) irreguardless of whether it is alive or not.

Paradoxical nocturnal dyspnea (PND) - sudden SOB while sleeping.

Parenteral – any medication route other than mouth.

Paresis – partial or incomplete paralysis.

Post prandially – after a meal.

Precocious – exceptionally early in development or occurance; mature qualities at an early age

Priapism – abnormal, painful, and continued erection of the penis caused by disease, occurring usually without sexual desire.

Primigravida – a women during her first pregnancy.

Primipara – a women who has delivered of one infant of 500g (or 20weeks), reguardless of it's viability.

Primum non nocere – first do no harm.

Procidentia – complete prolapse, especially of the uterus, to such anextent that the uterus lies outside of the vulva with everted vaginal walls.

Prognosticate – to fortell from signs & symptoms; predict.

Proscription – behavior that is forbidden by religious or cultural tenet of belief.

Pruritis – severe itching.

Quickening – first movements of the fetus felt in utero usually by the 18th -20th week (rare by 10th wk).

Psychosis – a disturbance of such magnitude that there is personality disintegration and loss of contact with reality usually characterized by delusions and hallucinations.

Recalcitrant - usually not responsive to treatment.

Recrudescent – assuming renewed activity after a dormant or inactive period.

Refractory – resistant to ordinary treatment.

Satyriasis – excessive or abnormal sexual craving in the male (see nymphomania).

Scintillations - luminous wavy patch in visual field.

Scotmas - island like blind spot in visual field.

Senescence – the state or process of becoming old.

Sialorrhea – excessive secretion of saliva.

Somnolence – prolonged drowsiness or a condition resembling a trance that may continue for a number of days; sleepiness.

Spasticity – increased tone or contractions of muscles causing stiffness and awkward movements; the result of an upper motor neuronal lesion.

Striae gravidarum – a fine pinkish-white or gray line, usu seen in parts of the body where skin has been stretched (thighs, abdomen, breasts).

Succinct – marked by compact precise expression without wasted words; syn concise

Superfluous – exceeding what is sufficient or necessary; marked by wastefulness.

Synesthesias – a sensory stimulus producing a perception in a differenct sensory modality, e.g., seeing sound.

Teichopsia – scintillating scotoma in eyes usually associated with migranes.

Tenesmus – spasmodic contraction of anal or bladder sphincter with pain & persistent desire to empty the bowel or bladder with involuntary ineffectual straining efforts.

Thrombophlebitis - thrombus causing inflamation of a vein.

Tinnitus - ringing in ears.

Tropism – involuntary orientation by an organisim or one of its parts that involves turning or curving by movement or by differential growth and is a positive or negative response to a source of stimulation. (e.g., how some types of viruses always seems to only attack the upper respiratory track).

Undulant – rise and fall like waves (like an undulating fever).

Volition – an act of making a choice or decision.

Notes

Abbreviations:

Medical professionals use abbreviations as though they are words in the English language. Unfortunately for the medical student, many early mornings are spent trying to understand these esoteric scripts in SOAP notes (never mind trying to decipher the cryptic handwriting). Although difficult to master initially, they are a real time saver once you start to use them in your notes and H&Ps. I would recommend to simply look them up as you encounter them – don't try to memorize this list. The following are commonly used abbreviations (some are illegal to use):

° - hour
Δ - change
Ψ - Psych (as is order a psych evaluation for this patient)
↓ - decrease
↑ - increase
♀ - female
♂ - male
a - (with a line over): before
p - (with a line over): after
c - (with a line over): with
s - (with a line over): without
A+O x 3 - "alert and oriented x 3 (to time, place, person)"
A-a - Alveolar Arterial gradient
AA - Alcoholics Anonymous; African American
AAA - abdominal aortic aneurysm.
Ab Antibody, Abortion
ABD - Abdomen
ABE - acute bacterial endocarditis
ABG - arterial blood gas
ABI - Ankle Brachial Index
ABX - Antibiotics
ACE-I - Angiotensin Converting Enzyme Inhibitor
ACL - Anterior Cruciate Ligament
ACLS - Advanced Cardiac Life Support
ACS - Acute Coronary Syndrome
AD LIB - As Desired
ADA - American Diabetes Association
ADD - Attention Deficit Disorder
ADE - Adverse Drug Effect
ADH - antidiuretic hormone
ADHD - Attention Deficit Hyperactivity Disorder
AED - Automatic External Defibrillator; Anti-Epileptic Drug
AF - Atrial Fibrillation; Afebrile
AFB - acid-fast bacillus (TB)
AFP - alpha-fetoprotein
Ag - Antigen
AI - aortic insufficiency
AIDS - Acquired Immuno-Deficiency Syndrome

AKA - above knee amputation
ALL - acute lymphocytic leukemia
ALS - amyotropic lateral sclerosis
ALT - alanine aminotransferase (same as SGPT)
AMA - Against Medical Advice; American Medical Association
AMD - Aging Macular Degeneration
AMI - Acute Myocardial Infarction; Anterior Myocardial Infarction
AML - Acute Myelogenous Leukemia
ANC - Absolute Neutrophil Count
ANA - anti-nuclear antibody
ANGIO - Angiography
AP - Anterior-Posterior
A/P - Assessment and Plan
APC - Atrial Premature Contraction
APPY - Appendectomy
AR - aortic regurgitation
ARDS - Adult Respiratory Distress Syndrome
ARF - acute renal failure
AS - aortic stenosis
ASA - aspirin
ASD - atrial septal defect
AST - aspartic aminotransferase (same as SGOT)
ATN - acute tubular necrosis
AVM - arteriovenous malformation
AVR - aortic valve replacement
A/V Nicking - Arteriolar/Venous Nicking
A/V Ratio - Arteriolar/Venous Ratio
AVF- Arterio-Venous Fistula
AVN - Avascular Necrosis
AVNRT - Atrio-Ventricular Nodal Reentrant Tachycardia
AVR - Aortic Valve Replacment
AVSS - Afebrile, Vital Signs Stable
B - Bilateral
BBB - Bundle Branch Block
BCC - Basal Cell Carcinoma
BCG - Bacille Calmette-Guerin
B CX - Blood Culture
BE - Bacterial Endocarditis; also Barium Enema
BID - Twice a Day
BIPAP - Bi-Level Positive Airway Pressure

BIVAD - Bi-Ventricular Assist Device
BKA - Below Knee Amputation
BM - Bone Marrow; also Bowel Movement
BMI - Body Mass Index
BMT - Bone Marrow Transplant
BP - Blood Pressure
BPD - Borderline Personality Disorder; also
Bi-Polar Disorder and
Broncho-Pulmonary Dysplasia
BPH - benign prostatic hypertrophy
BPM - beats per minute
BPV - Benign Positional Vertigo
BR - Bed Rest
BRB - Bright Red Blood
BRBPR - Bright Red Blood Per Rectum
BRP - Bathroom Priveleges
BS - Bowel Sounds; also Breath Sounds and
Blood Sugar
BSA - Body Surface Area
BSO - bilateral salpingo-oophorectomy
BUN - Blood Urea Nitrogen
Bx - Biopsy
c (the letter with a line over) - With
C - chills or constipation
C&S - culture and sensitivity
Ca cancer, calcium
CABG - Coronary Artery By-Pass Graft
CAD - Coronary Artery Disease
CAP - Prostate Cancer; Community Acquired
Pneumonia
CAPD - continual ambulatory peritoneal
dialysis
CAT - Cataract
CATH - Catheterization
CB - Cerebellar
CBC - Complete Blood Count
CBD - Common Bile Duct; Closed Bag
Drainage
cc - Chief Complaint
CCB - Calcium Channel Blocker
C/C/E - clubbing, cyanosis, edema
CCK - Cholycystectomy
CCU - coronary care unit
C/D - Cup to Disk ratio
CDI - Clean Dry Intact
C DIF - Clostridium Difficile
CEA - Carcinoembryonic Antigen
CF - cystic fibrosis
Chemo - Chemotherapy
CHI - Closed Head Injury
CHF - Congestive Heart Failure
Choly - Cholycystectomy
CI - Cardiac Index
CIN - cervical intraepithelial neoplasia
cis - carcinoma in situ

CK - Creatine Kinase
CLL - Chronic Lymphocytic Leukemia
CM - Cardiomegaly
CML - Chronic Myelogenous Leukemia
CMT - Cervical Motion Tenderness; Charcot
Marie Tooth
CMV - Cytomegalovirus
CN - Cranial Nerves
CNS - Central Nervous System
CO - Cardiac Output
c/o - Complains Of
COPD - Chronic Obtructive Pulmonary
Disease
COX 2 - Cyclooxygenase 2
CP - chest pain
CPAP - Continuous Positive Airway Pressure
CPK;CK - creatinine phosphokinase
CPR - Cardiopulmonary Recusitation
CPS - Child Protective Services
CRF - Chronic renal failure
CRI - Chronic Renal Insufficiency
CRP - C Reactive Protein
CSF - Cerebral Spinal Fluid
CT - Cat Scan; also Chest Tube and Cardio-
Thoracic
CTA - Clear To Auscultation
CVA - costovertebral angle; cerebrovascular
accident
CVL - Central Venous Line
CVP - Central Venous Pressure
CX - Culture or chest
CXR - Chest X-Ray
C/W - Consistent With
D - Diarrhea; also Disk
D5LR - dextrose 5% in lactated ringer's
solution
D5NS - dextrose 5% in normal saline
D5W - Dextrose 5% in Water
DA - dopamine
DB - Direct Bilirubin
DBP - Diastolic Blood Pressure
DC - Discharge; Discontinue; Doctor of
Chiropractics
D&C - Dilatation and Curretage
DCIS - Ductal Carcinoma In Situ
ddx - Differential Diagnosis
DFA - Direct Flourescent Antibody
DI - Diabetes Insipidus; Detrusor Instability
DIC - Disseminated Intravascular
Coagulopathy
DIF - Differential
DIP - Distal Inter-Phalangeal (joint)
DJD - Degenerative Joint Disease
DKA - Diabetic Ketoacidosis
DM - Diabetes Mellitus

90

DNI - Do Not Intubate
DNR - Do Not Recusitate (keep doing what your doing, just don't do extra)
DOA - dead on arrival
DO - Doctor of Osteopahty
DOE - dyspnea on exertion
DP - Dorsalis Pedis
DPL - Diagnostic Peritoneal Lavage
DRE - Digital Rectal Exam
DTs - Delirium Tremens
DTR - Deep Tendon Reflex
DTP - diptheria, tetanus toxoid, pertussis vaccine
DVT - Deep Venous Thrombosis
DX - Diagnosis
DU - Duodenal Ulcer
DZ - disease
EBL - Estimated Blood Loss
EBRT - External Beam Radiation Therapy
EBV - Epstein Barr Virus
ECG - Electrocardiogram (also known as EKG)
ECMO - Extra-Corporeal Membrane Oxygenation
ECT - Electro-Convulsive Therapy
ED - Errectile Dysfunction
EDC - expected date of confinement (i.e., date of delivery of baby)
EEG - Electroencephalogram
EF - Ejection Fraction (in reference to ventricular function)
EGD - Esophago-Gastro Duodenoscopy
EJ - External Jugular
EKG - Electrocardiogram (also known as ECG)
EM - Electron Microscopy
EMG - Electromyelogram
EMS - Emergency Medical System
EMT - Emergency Medical Technician
EOMI - Extra Occular Muscles Intact
Eos - Eosinophils
EPO - Erythropoeitin
EPS - Electro-Physiologic Study
ER - External Rotation; also Emergency Room
ERCP - Endoscopic Retrograde Cholangio-Pancreotography
ES - Epidural Steroids
ESLD - End Stage Liver Disease
ESR - Erythrocyte Sedimentation Rate
ESRD - End Stage Renal Disease
ESWL - Extracorporeal Shock Wave Lithotripsy
ETOH - Alcohol
ETT - Endotracheal Tube
EX LAP - Exploratory Laparotomy

EX FIX - External Fixation
EXT - Extremities
F - Fever
FB - Foreign Body
FBS - Fasting Blood Sugar
FE - Iron
FEM - Femoral
FENA - Fractional Excretion of Sodium
FEF - forced expiratory flow
FEV1 - Forced Expiratory Volume 1 Second
FFP - Fresh Frozen Plasma
FH - family history
FiO2 - fraction of inspired oxygen
Flex Sig - Flexible Sigmoidoscopy
FLU - Influenza
FMG - Foreign Medical Graduate
FNA - Fine Needle Aspiration
FP - Family Practitioner
FRC - Functional Residual Capacity
FROM – Full range of motion
FSG - Finger Stick Glucose
FSH - Follicle Stimulating Hormone
FTA-ABS flourescent treponemal antibody absorption (syphilis)
FTN - finger-to-nose
FTT - Failure To Thrive
F/U - Follow-Up
FUO - Fever of Unknown Origin
FVC - forced vital capacity
fx - Fracture
G - Guiac (followed by + or -)
GA - General Anesthesia
GAD - Generalized Anxiety Disorder
GAS - Group A Strep
GB - Gall Bladder; also Guillain Barre
GBM - Glioblastoma Multiforme
GBS - Group B Strep
GC - Gonorrhea
GCS - Glascow Coma Scale
GCSF - Granulocyte Colony Stimulating Factor
GERD - Gastroesophageal Reflux
GERI- Geriatrics
GI - Gastrointestinal
GNR - Gram Negative Rod
GP - General Practitioner
G#P# - Gravida # Para # (pregnancies, deliveries)
GP 2b/3a - Glycoprotein 2b/3a Inhibitor
GPC - Gram Positive Coccus
GS - Gram Stain
GSW - Gun Shot Wound
GTT - Glucose Tolerance Test or gtts=drips
G-Tube - Gastric Feeding Tube

GU - Genito-Urinary; also Gastric Ulcer
GVHD - Graft Versus Host Disease
H FLU - Haemophilus Influenza
H2 - Histamine 2
HA - Headache
HAART - Highly Active Anti-Retroviral Therapy
HAV - hepatitis A virus
HBcAg - hepatitis B core antigen
HBIG - hepatitis B immune globulin
HBsAg - hepatitis B surface antigen
HCC - Hepatocellular Carcinoma
HCG - Human Chorionic Gonadotropin
HCT - Hematocrit
HCTZ - hydrochlorothiazide
HCV - Hepatitis C Virus
HD - Hemodialysis, hospital day 0, Hodgkin's disease
HDL - High Density Lipoprotein
HEENT - Head, Ears, Eyes, Nose, Throat
HELLP - Hemolysis Elevated Liver tests Low Platelets
HEME/ONC - Hematology/Oncology
HGB - Hemoglobin
H&H - Hemoglobin and Hematocrit
HI - Homicidal Ideation
HIB - Haemophilus Influenza B vaccine
HIT - Heparin Induced Thrombocytopenia
HIV - Human Immunodeficiency Virus
HJR - hepatojugular reflex
HLA - histocompatibility locus antigen
h/o - history of
HO- house officer
HOB - Head Of Bed
HOCM - Hypertrophic Obstructive Cardiomyopathy
HPI - History of Present Illness
HPL - human placental lactogen
HPV - Human Papilloma Virus
HR - Heart Rate
HRT - Hormone Replacement Therapy
hs - At Bedtime
HSP - Henoch Shonlein Purpura
HSV - Herpes Simplex Virus
HTN - Hypertension
HUS - Hemolytic Uremic Syndrome
HX - History
IABP - Intra-Aortic Baloon Pump
IBD - Inflammatory Bowel Disease
IBS - Irritable Bowel Syndrome
IBW - Ideal Body Weight
ICD - Implantable Cardiac Defibrillator
ICP - Intra-Cranial Pressure
ID - Infectious Diseases
I&D - Incise and Drain

IDDM - Insulin Dependent Diabetes Mellitus
IFN - Interferon
IHSS - Idiopathic hypertrophic subaortic stenosis
IJ - Internal Jugular
IL- Interleukin; Indirect Layngoscopy
IM - Intramuscular also Intramedullary
IMP - Impression
imv - intermittent minute ventilation
INH - isoniazid
INR - International Normalized Ratio
I&O - Ins and Outs
IOP - Intra-Occular Pressure
IP - Inter-Phalangeal
IR - Interventional Radiology
IRB - Institutional Review Board
IT - Intrathecal; Information Technology
ITP - Idiopathic Thrombocytopenia
IUD - Intrauterine Device
IUGR - intrauterine growth retardation
IUP - Intrauterine Pregnancy
IV - Intravenous
IVC - Inferior Vena Cava
IVDU - Intravenous Drug Use
IVF - Intravenous Fluids; also In Vitro Fertilization
IVP - Intravenous Pyelogram
JP - Jackson Pratt (a type of drain)
J-Tube - Jejunal Feeding Tube
JVD - Jugular Venous Distention
JVP - Jugular Venous Pressure
K - Potassium
KCl - potassium chloride
KCAL - Kilocalories
KUB - Kidneys Ureters and Bladder (X-ray of abdomen area looking at these)
KVO - Keep Vein Open
L - Left
LA - Left Atrium
LAC - Laceration
LAD - Left Anterior Descending (coronary artery); Left Axis Deviation
LAP - Laproscopic; also Laparotomy
LBBB - Left Bundle Branch Block
LCL - Lateral Collateral Ligament
LCX - Left Circumflex (coronary artery)
LD - lethal dose; loading dose; lactate dehydrogenase
L&D - Labor and Delivery
LDH - Lactate Dehydrogenase
LDL - Low Density Lipoprotein
LE - Lower Extremity (usually preceded by R or L); Leukocyte Esterase
LFT - Liver Function Test
LH - Leutinizing Hormone; Left Handed;

Light Headed
LHRH - Leutinizing Hormone Releasing Hormone
LLE- Left Lower Extremity
LLL - Left Lower Lobe; Left Lower Lid
LLQ - Left Lower Quadrant
LMP - last menstrual period (first day of the LMP)
LOA - Lysis Of Adhesions, left occiput anterior
LOC - Loss Of Consciousness
LP - Lumbar Puncture
LPN - Licensed Practical Nurse
LR - Lactated Ringers (an IV solution)
L/S - ratio lecithin/sphingomyelin ratio
LUE - Left Upper Extremity
LUQ - Left Upper Quadrant
LVEDP - left ventricular end diastolic pressure
LVEDV - left ventricular end diastolic volume
LV FXN - Left Ventricular Function
LVEDP - Left Ventricular End Diastolic Pressure
LVH - Left Ventricular Hypertrophy
LYTES- Electrolytes
m - murmur
mai - mycobacterium avium-intracellularae
MAC - Monitored Anesthesia Care, minimum alveolar concentration
MAO - monoamine oxidase
MAP - mean aortic pressure
MAST - military antishock trousers
MCH - mean corpuscular hemoglobin
MCHC - mean corpuscular hemoglobin concentration
MCL - Medial Collateral Ligament
MCP - Metacarpal-Phalangeal joint
MCV - Mean Corpuscular Volume
MEDS - Medicines
Mets - metastases
MgSO4 - magnesium sulfate
MI - Myocardial Infarction
MICU - Medical Intensive Care Unit
M&M - Morbidity and Mortality
MMR - Measels, Mumps and Rubella vaccine
MOM - Milk Of Magnesia
MR - mental retardation; metabolic rate; mitral regurgitation;
MRCP - Magnetic Resonance Cholangio Pancreatography
MRI - Magnetic Resonance Imaging
MRSA - Methicillin Resistant Staph Aureus
MS - Mental Status; also Mitral Stenosis, Multiple Sclerosis and Morphine Sulfate
MSE - mental status exam
MSO4 - Morphine Sulfate

MSSA - Methicillin Sensitive Staph Aureus
MVA - motor vehicle accident
MVP - Mitral Valve Prolapse
MVR - Mitral Valve Replacement
N - Nausea
NA - Not Available; also Sodium
NAD - No Apparent Distress
nc - nasal cannula
nd - non-distended
NEB - Nebulizer
NGT - Naso-Gastric Tube
NH - Nursing Home
NHL - Non-Hodgkin's Lymphoma
NICU - Neonatal Intensive Care Unit
NIDDM - Non-Insulin Dependent Diabetes Mellitus
NKDA - No Known Drug Allergies
NMS - Neuroleptic Malignant Syndrome
NOS - Not Otherwise Specified
NP - Nurse Practitioner
NPH - normal pressure hydrocephalus
NPO - Nothing By Mouth
NS - Normal Saline
NSAID - non-steroidal anti-inflammatory
NSCLCA - Non-Small Cell Lung Cancer
NSR - Normal Sinus Rhythm
NSVD - normal spontaneous vaginal delivery
NSSTTW's - nonspecific ST, T wave changes
nt - nontender; nasotracheal
NT – non tender
NTD - Nothing To Do
NTG - nitroglycerin
nt/nd - nontender, nondistended
NUCS - Nuclear Medicine
N/V/F/C - nausea, vomiting, fever, chills
Ox3 - oriented to person, place, and time ("times 3")
OA - Osteoarthritis
OCD - Obsessive Compulsive Disorder
OCP - Oral Contraceptive Pill
OD - Right Eye, overdose
OOB - Out Of Bed
O&P - Ovum and Parasistes
OPV - oral polio vaccine
OR - operating room
ORIF - Open Reduction with Internal Fixation
ORL - Oto-Rhino Laryngology
OS - Left Eye
OT - Occupational Therapy
OTC - Over The Counter
OTD - Out The Door
O/W - Otherwise
P – Pulse, Pending
p (with a line over) - After
PA - Posterior-Anterior; also Physician's

Assistant
PAD - Peripheral Arterial Disease
PALS - Pediatric Advanced Life Support
Pap - Papanicolaou (vaginal smear for cancer)
PC - After Meals
PCA - Patient Controled Analgesia
PCI - Percutaneous Coronary Intervention
PCKD - Polycystic Kidney Disease
PCL - Posterior Cruciate Ligament
PCN - penicillin
PCP - Primary Care Physician; also
Pneumocystis Pneumonia
PCR - Polymerase Chain Reaction
PCWP - Pulmonary Capillary Wedge Pressure
PCXR - portable chest x-ray
PD - Parkinson's Disease; also Personality
Disorder and Peritoneal Dialysis
PDA - Patent Ductus Arteriosus
PE - physical exam; pulmonary embolism or
pulmonary edema; pleural effusion
PEEP - positive end expiratory pressure
PEG - Percutaneous Endoscopic Gastrostomy
PERRL - pupils equal, round, reactive to light
PERRLA - pupils equal, round, reactive to
light and accomodation
PET - Positron Emission Tomography
PF - Peak Flow
PFO - Patent Foramen Ovale
PFTs - Pulmonary Function Tests
PICA - posterior inferior cerebellar artery
PICC - Peripherally Inserted Central Catheter
PICU - Pediatric Intensive Care Unit
PID - Pelvic Inflammatory Disease
PIP - Proximal Inter-Phalangeal (joint)
PKU - phenylketonuria
PLT - Platelets
PMH - Past Medical History
PMI - Point of Maximum Impulse
PMN - Polymorphonuclear Leukocytes
PN - Progress Note
PND - Paroxysmal Nocturnal Dyspnea also
Post Nasal Drip
PNS - Peripheral Nervous System
PO - By Mouth
POD - post-operative day
POP - Popliteal
pp - post-prandial
PPD - Purified Protein Derivative
PPI - Proton Pump Inhibitor
PPN - Peripheral Parenteral Nutrition
PR - Per Rectum
PRBCs - Packed Red Blood Cells
PRN - Refers to treatments which patient can
receive on an "as needed" basis
PROM - premature rupture of membranes

PSA - Prostate Specific Antigen
PSC - Primary Sclerosing Cholangitis
PSH - Past Surgical History
PT - Physical Therapy; Posterior Tibial;
Prothrombin Time; Patient
PTCA - Percutaneous Transluminal Coronary
Angioplasty
PTH - parathyroid hormone
P-Thal - Persantine Thallium
pt - patient
PTSD - Post-Traumatic Stress Disorder
PTT - Partial Thromboplastin Time
PTX - Pneumothorax
PUD - Peptic Ulcer Disease
P VAX - Pneumococcal Vaccination
PVC - Premature Ventricular Contraction
PVD - Peripheral Vascular Disease; Posterior
Vitreous Detachment
PWP - pulmonary wedge pressure
Q6 – every 6 hrs
QAM - each morning
QD – every day
QHS - every night
QID - four times per day
QM - every month
QOD - every other day
QPM - each evening
QW – every week
R - Right
RA - rheumatoid arthritis; right atrium
RAD - Right Axis Deviation; also Reactive
Airways Disease
RAE - right atrial enlargement
RBBB - Right Bundle Branch Block
RBC - Red Blood Cell
RCA - Right Coronary Artery
RDA - recommended daily allowance
RF - Rheumatoid Factor; also Risk Factor
RHD - Rheumatic Heart Disease
Rheum - Rheumatology
RLE - Right Lower Extremity
RLL - Right Lower Lobe
RLQ - Right Lower Quadrant
R/O - Rule Out
ROM - Range Of Motion, rupture of
membranes
ROS - Review Of Systems
RPGN - Rapidly Progressive
Glomerulonephritis
RPR - rapid plasma reagin (test for syphilis)
RR - Respiratory Rate
RRR - Regular Rate and Rhythm
RSD - Reflex Sympathetic Dystrophy
RSV - Respiratory Syncytial Virus

RT - Respiratory Therapy
RTA - renal tubular acidosis
RTC - Return To Clinic
RUE - Right Upper Extremity
RUQ - Right Upper Quadrant
RV - Right Ventricle; Residual Volume
RVH - right ventricle hypertrophy
RVR- Rapid Ventricular Response
RX – Treatment, prescription pharmaceuticals
RXN - reaction
S (with a line over)- Without
SA - Sino-Atrial; Staph Aureus
SAH - Sub-Arachnoid Hemorrhage
SBE - Subacute Bacterial Endocarditis
SBO - Small Bowel Obstruction
SBP - Spontaneous Bacterial Peritonitis;
Systolic Blood Pressure
SC - Subcutaneous
SCLCA - Small Cell Lung Cancer
SFA - Superficial Femoral Artery
SFV - Superficial Femoral Vein
SGOT - serum glutamic oxaloacetic
transaminase (same as AST)
SGPT - serum glutamic pyruvic transaminase
(same as ALT)
SI - Suicidal Ideation or small intestine (SI/HI
suicidal ideation/homicidal ideation)
SIADH - Syndrome of Inappropriate Anti-
Diuretic Hormone secretion
SICU - Surgical Intensive Care Unit
SIDS - Sudden Infant Death Syndrome
Sig: indicating instructions to take medicine as
follows ("signa")
SIRS - Systemic Inflammatory Response
Syndrome
SL - Sublingual
SLE - Systemic Lupus Erythematosus; also
Slit Lamp Exam
SOB shortness of breath
S/P - status post (e.g., S/P cardiac arrest, S/P
hysterectomy, etc.)
SPF - Sun Protection Formula
SROM - spontaneous rupture of membranes
SQ - Subcutaneous
SSI - Sliding Scale Insulin
SSPE - subacute sclerosing panencephalitis
SSRI - Selective Serotonin Reuptake Inhibitor
STAT - Immediately
STD - Sexually Transmitted Disease
SV - stroke volume; supraventricular
SVC - Superior Vena Cava
SVG - Saphenous Vein Graft
SVT - supraventricular tachycardia
SX - Symptoms
SZ - Seizure

T - Temperature
TAH/BSO - total abdominal
hysterectomy/bilateral
salpingoophorectomy
TB - Tuberculosis; Total Bilirubin
TBG - thyroxine binding globulin
TBW - total body weight; total body water
T&C - Type and Cross
TCA - Tricyclic Antidepressant
TD - Tetanus and Diptheria Vaccination;
Tardive Dyskinesia
TEE - Trans-Esophageal Echocardiogram
TFs - Tube Feeds
TG - Triglycerides
TIA - Transient Ischemic Attack
TIBC - Total Iron Binding Capacity
TID - Three times per day
TIPS - Transvenous Intrahepatic Porto-
Systemic Shunt
TKA - Total Knee Arthroplasty
TKO - to keep open (IV at a slow rate)
TM - Tympanic Membrane
Tmax - highest temperature (usually within
last 24 hours)
TMJ - Temporo-Mandibular Joint
TMN - Tumor Metastases Nodes (universal
tumor staging system)
TNF - Tumor Necrosis Factor
TOA - Tubo-Ovarian Abscess
TOPV - trivalent oral polio vaccine
TOX - Toxicology
TOXO - Toxoplasmosis
TP - Total Protein
TPA - Tissue Plasminogen Activator
TPN - Total Parenteral Nutrition
T-PTX - tension pneumothorax
TR - Tricuspid Regurgitation
T&S - Type and Screen
TS - tricuspid stenosis
TSH - Thyroid Stimulating Hormone
TSS - toxic shock syndrome
TTE - Trans-Thoracic Echocardiogram
TTP - Thrombotic Thrombocytopenic Purpura
TURP - Transurethral Prostatectomy
TV - Tidal Volume
TX - Transfusion; Treatment; transplant
u - units (as in Insulin)
UA - Urine Analysis; also Uric Acid
UC - Ulcerative Colitis
UCX - Urine Culture
UE - Upper Extremity (usu with R or L)
URI - Upper Respiratory tract Infection
U/S, US - Ultrasound
UTI - Urinary Tract Infection
V - Vomiting

VBAC - Vaginal Birth After Cesearean Section
VC - Vital Capacity
VD - venereal disease
VDRL - syphilis test (stands for "Venereal Disease Research Laboratory")
VF - Ventricular Fibrillation
VIP - Vasoactive Intestinal Peptide
VLDL - very low density lipoprotein
VMA - vanillymandelic acid
VS - Vital Signs
VSD - Ventricular Septal Defect
VSS - Vital Signs Stable
VT - Ventricular Tachycardia
VWF - Von Willebrand Factor
VZV - varicella zoster virus
WBC - White Blood Cells
WDWN - Well Developed, Well Nourished
WNL - Within Normal Limits; we never looked
W/O - Without
WPW - Wolff-Parkinson-White syndrome
X - Except
XRT - Radiation Therapy
yo - years old

Notes